The Palgrave Lacan Series

Jacques Lacan is one of the most important and influential thinkers of the 20th century. The reach of this influence continues to grow as we settle into the 21st century, the resonance of Lacan's thought arguably only beginning now to be properly felt, both in terms of its application to clinical matters and in its application to a range of human activities and interests. The Palgrave Lacan Series is a book series for the best new writing in the Lacanian field, giving voice to the leading writers of a new generation of Lacanian thought. The series will comprise original monographs and thematic, multi-authored collections. The books in the series will explore aspects of Lacan's theory from new perspectives and with original insights. There will be books focused on particular areas of or issues in clinical work. There will be books focused on applying Lacanian theory to areas and issues beyond the clinic, to matters of society, politics, the arts and culture. Each book, whatever its particular concern, will work to expand our understanding of Lacan's theory and its value in the 21st century.

Sheila L. Cavanagh

Bracha L. Ettinger and Jacques Lacan

Psychoanalysis, Sexuality, and the m/Other

palgrave
macmillan

Sheila L. Cavanagh
Sociology
York University
Toronto, ON, Canada

ISSN 2946-4196 ISSN 2946-420X (electronic)
The Palgrave Lacan Series
ISBN 978-3-032-23292-2 ISBN 978-3-032-23293-9 (eBook)
https://doi.org/10.1007/978-3-032-23293-9

This work was supported by Social Sciences and Humanities Research Council of Canada.

This Palgrave Macmillan imprint is published by the registered company Springer Nature Switzerland AG.
The registered company address is: Gewerbestrasse 11, 6330 Cham, Switzerland

Foreword

As a reader of psychoanalysis, there must come a certain moment when the field's overwhelming misogyny is felt, one directed the most vehemently at mothers. There is very little that a mother can do right—she is always too much, or too little, her hate is shattering, and her failures and defects are responsible for everything broken in a child, meaning mothers are the place we lodge our blame for what is wrong with the world. Erik Erikson in his esteemed work "Childhood and Society" from 1952 asks how blaming mothers for all psychopathology became a literary sport of acceptable temper tantrums by an entire field. Later, the psychoanalyst Bracha L. Ettinger called this endemic problem in mental health "the ready-made Mother monster." I sometimes wonder as a woman and a mother how I've stayed so invested in psychoanalysis.

This book by Sheila Cavanagh is long overdue. Placing Bracha L Ettinger's work within the wider context of psychoanalysis and its systems, we begin to sense the possibility for another model, another way of working, beginning with the mother and the feminine. The failure to think women, mothers, intrauterine life, birth, and pro-creation, which would seem fundamentally tied to psychic capacities of linkage, connection, relation, and creativity, means psychoanalysis takes these capacities and attributes them to men, fathers, and their role in the establishment of society and culture. So, a woman is she who either "does not exist" or whose existence is too overwhelming. A woman or mother requires the father's restrictions, by name and by law, for the continued order of a given culture and its innocent children. Finally, with this contextualization of Bracha's work, we can clearly see the possibility of doing it the other way round, something that some psychoanalysts said would be "regressive." Cavanagh shows that this reversal might be the most progressive and interesting version of psychoanalysis available to us, one that Bracha has been working on for decades and decades now.

Cavanagh's book offers one of the clearest engagements with Bracha's thought from within the field of Lacanian psychoanalysis. Cavanagh shows how Ettinger's matrixial reframes familiar clinical and literary objects without abandoning Lacan, but by reading him from another axis—one that already made gestures of returning the mother, the feminine, and intrauterine life to the heart of psychoanalytic theory. This book stands apart for the way it refuses the false choice so often imposed on readers—Ettinger *or* Lacan, feminism *or* psychoanalysis—and instead demonstrates how the matrixial supplements, challenges, and ultimately expands the Lacanian field. It is a book that both situates Ettinger historically and allows her thought to breathe within clinical cases and texts that have long been read through a narrower optic. If the reader is new to the matrixial, this volume is a guide; if they are wary of Ettinger because Lacanian discourse has taught them to be, this book opens the door.

*

Allow me a little digression: At a certain point in one's career as a psychoanalyst, transference becomes a rare and longed for feeling. Constantly in the position of negotiating the transference of others, one struggles to muster that great and passionate illusion for oneself. Bracha L. Ettinger is one of my last teachers—one of the few figures whose work continues to produce transference rather than mastery. I've had a sense for some time that she knows something very precious and particular about the most obscure and complex aspects of psychoanalytic work involving the question of the Mother, women, and negotiating sexual difference without giving up relation, which she investigates not only in her self-analysis and work with patients, but in her art and psychoanalytic theory. She is the only psychoanalyst I know who is also an artist continually exhibiting in galleries and museums across the world. Her work is true praxis in the sense of putting ideas to work.

Having had a daughter recently, the encounter with Bracha's work has been vital to my life once again since the first time I learned of her in my early twenties. In particular, I'm interested in the amortization rate of a woman's bodily life stretched between birth, menstruation, pregnancy, and motherhood, and the losses that these continually entail in a patriarchal world. Her work on "the matrixial," a concept that she has been working on since the 1980s, is a powerful rewriting of Lacan, as she would put it, from the Other direction. Instead of the Other always being what is negotiated, denied, severed, and finally repudiated by an identitarian world, we might write from the sense of connection to the Other, and the ways in which she is lost to us but yet we maintain a connection somewhere.

Women, Bracha says, are the carriers of the "wound-spaces" of human life. How to listen to this is the difficult task of the analyst, not because one doesn't want to hear about it (perhaps one doesn't), but because it is effectively buried by civilization, discourse, and cognition. *Traum*, or dream in German, resonates strongly with trauma, or wound, and space in Hebrew, חלל *(halal)* can also be translated as wound or cavity. The link between what opens, or what is open, to what is wounding, unconscious, part of the network that is dream life, is perhaps one of the most basic psychoanalytic problems—the difficulty of going *there*.

I had a first dream about my daughter, Alma, in her infancy, which was somehow also about psychoanalysis. I was with another teacher of mine, a child psychoanalyst, and we were singing karaoke. Older now, in the dream he was in full glory. The scene then switched and I had fallen asleep and Alma had gotten ahold of something in bed. I rushed to her and she had eaten a bunch of fishing line. I pulled it out of her mouth, a process which felt endless; the line was practically infinite, and along the way there was the occasional hook, which frightened me, though she seemed to be ok. Pulling out these threads—which felt as if they came from the deepest part of her, as if they transcended the small confines of her body—I wondered if she was damaged by all this. And then I woke up. What frightened me was not only the danger to her but also the sense that meaning itself arrived as something threaded, resistant to extraction, and never entirely my own.

After Alma emerged from the newborn phase, she emerged as a voice—loud, powerful, almost a song. Where did this come from? Where had she been those first three months, lost to the trauma of birth? And where is this joy in sound on the edge of language in the rest of us? Her precocious voice left me with these questions. Bracha quotes Paul Celan in her paper on the concept of "carriance": "THREAD SUNS / above the grey-black wilderness [–]/ there are / still songs to be sung on the other side / of mankind." Carrying, she says, is its own kind of knowledge, a learning that is mostly unconscious, and emerges in what she calls threads, string-working; for even if we are in withdrawal from others and the world, "webbing continues. Nets are knotted." "At what depth?" she asks. Answering: the depth where having hurt the other, it hurts in us, reverberating across these living strings. Alma means soul, learned, world. Alma Mater.

Matrixial sublimation happens at the periphery of language and image, not entirely separate from them, requiring what Bracha might call experimental links at the border. Like Ariadne, the psychoanalyst follows these strings in the form of listening that we practice, and we have to experiment with speaking to what we hear. We reach past individuals to something transindividual; we reach past reality, to something she calls the subreal. We might name this the intergenerational transmission of trauma which cuts across the pathos of our individually experienced pain. We might also call this creativity—what we know beyond the conscious constraints of what we are allowed to know. This is, in my field, blithely called "interpretation," which hardly captures the act. One wonders if we might need an artist to render the art!

Many have also called this kind of work with the unconscious "mystical," meaning it reaches toward something ancient or ancestral in us, tapping into certain kinds of intuition beyond the senses. If this feels too grand or obscure to you, think of the pleasure in speaking without paying too much heed to sense, where the words and affects seem to rush out from under you, pushing the intensity of one's wit. I love when patients get closer to this. Freud, with his method of free association, wanted us to relax the watchman at the gates who wants to dictate what passes in accordance with the laws of reason and fact. It's a way of trying to remain separate, to not allow what is Other in us to come forth. To refuse to be carried away.

The matrixial thus speaks to a different kind of being with others. Bracha models this on the image of the infant in utero and the mother carrying the fetus to term, but also on much of what psychoanalysis has understood regarding childhood, the prolonged helplessness of human infants and the way they must be continually carried. As well, she recenters the importance of bi-sexuality in the Freudian model, meaning that what she names women is open to all. Bracha's theory is not essentialist, and in fact is important to the current debates on gender and the attacks that women and those identified as LGBTQ+ have suffered.

Importantly, this is not symbiosis, fusion, or enmeshment, which in any case is the problem of the neurotically individuated subject who has difficulty with leaving their boundaries behind and can only do so wholesale, in a kind of fantastical take-over. This is being together with our differences intact. Through strange advances in imaging, I know that my daughter loved sucking on her umbilical cord. It would have had a different pulsating rhythm to that of her own body. She also responded vigorously to the sound of voices, of which, given my being a psychoanalyst, there were many for her to listen to throughout her days. All the way back, the Other is already there.

In accessing the human beyond individuation, Bracha hopes for a capacity to create new forms of exchange. This is the risk taken between an artist and their audience. She writes:

> The pressure I feel to produce significance, not to only paint, is pressure of conscience—my understanding that human beings and mainly the female-mothers collapse under culture's pressure to convert their experiences into that which remains at far too great a symbolic distance from their deep experience of the soul. I named a "women-artist" any artist whose life and work traverse, express and create matrixial spaces.

Her paintings are small, creating a space of intimacy. The infinite process of working over fragile traces of light and color feels tender. Emotionally charged, mythical scenes seem to emerge from beneath this abstract screen. Only by seeing these images in person could I sense how they give one the feeling of practicing psychoanalysis, working with another space of possibility beyond what is presented to us by the world, by our families, by the constraints of representation; what we work with only begins to appear through touching this texture or webbing of life at the limit of ourselves.

I came across a remark in one of Bracha's artist notebooks that often accompany her artwork and are sometimes exhibited: "not only…describing subjectivity in terms of split and matricide, but also proscribing it…Heroic efforts of both matrixial sublimation and of symbolizing the trap/fish in the water." My father is a fisherman. As a young girl, I remember watching the process of hooking small fish through their lips, in order to catch larger fish, then digging out the hooks from deep in these bigger fishes' mouths. I remember the excitement around catching a fish that would fight hard, which often meant they swallowed hard—hook, line, and sinker.

I was ambivalent about learning how to fish, which is certainly a knowledge to be passed on, but one that felt like a knowledge for men. Of course, this picture is metaphorically rich—the fragility a young girl feels in her body, questions about sexuality, penetration, male enjoyment, the troubled waters of father-daughter relationships that seem to be encapsulated in the idiom "shooting fish in a barrel." The sea, the fish, the hook, the catch, runs like a primal scene, replete with impregnation, water-breaking, birth, but also the pain of the bonds of love—*to have their hooks in you.*

There is also something more specific than this metaphorical scene: My father's mother's family were immigrant fisherman from the north of Sweden to the Midwest, where they encountered no end of problems: the Great Depression, loss of their farm, miscarriages, rape, alcoholism, postpartum melancholia, and tragic deaths. An image of life lived well in nature—which was bountiful and giving—was a nostalgic fantasy of my father's that covered over these traumas; perhaps there was even a fantasy of mother as Mother Earth, differently violent, violent out of sheer necessity.

I wish my daughter didn't have to swallow all of this. But my work also wouldn't be what it is without it, and this is what I have to pass on. On all sides then, Bracha and her painting, me and my psychoanalyzing, my father and his fishing, Alma and her singing: "heroic efforts of both matrixial sublimation and of symbolizing the trap/fish in the water."

*

There are so many ethical and aesthetic lessons to be learned from psychoanalysis once it begins with the question of the matrixial. Through Cavanagh's explorations of her work, especially in the female figures important to Bracha—Dora, Persephone, Duras, Antigone, Medea—we begin to have another language, maybe even another kind of language (less phallically burdened), to speak to the conundrums of life and suffering. What is speaking of suffering if it can have no resonance with the lived experience of being a woman, having a mother, being a mother, experiencing something beyond what is currently declared to be possible under patriarchy. I think of Bracha's work as an extension, not a detraction from Freud and Lacan, and importantly she leans on others: Deleuze and Guattari, Laing, and Winnicott. For those who know Lacan well, reading her will feel like second skin, with a few hooks removed and a thousand threads added.

We have needed Shelia Cavanagh's important book, a scholarly synthesis of Bracha's contributions and their stakes, a guide to reading her reworking of Lacan's framework, and a map of her various theories over time, which have spanned so many diverse audiences and contexts. Bracha writes for all: from academia, to the psychoanalytic clinic, to ethical studies and feminism, and finally aesthetics and the art world. Here we have a way into her work that centers the question of the matrixial, along with the difficulty for those who touch the feminine, the not-all, and must find a way to be. What distinguishes this book is not only its scholarly command, but its insistence that Ettinger's work must be read with Lacan rather than against him—a wager that changes the stakes of both.

Searching for what is beyond the phallic metonymy, language and reality coded patriarchal, and sexual difference that isn't reducible to male and its Other—Bracha teaches us to listen to these traces, threads, and webs. Cavanagh writes in a moment when sexual difference is either rigidly policed or prematurely dissolved, meaning this book offers a third position: one that insists on difference without violence and relation without fusion. Again, these impasses are too often encoded in masculine-phallic fantasies. We are being asked to accept a responsibility: to listen differently, to tolerate forms of knowing that do not arrive whole, and to remain answerable to what exceeds the individual subject. Cavanagh helps us do precisely that. You, readers, are in good hands to carry Bracha's work.

New York City, NY, USA Jamieson Webster

Acknowledgements

Writing a book is an exercise in self-discipline and time, but it is enabled by many people who support the process behind the scenes.

I am indebted to those who offered friendship, collegial support, editorial, and scholarly expertise. It took me over ten years to write this book, in part, because Bracha's work demands attention to the mother. Although my book is not autobiographical, matrixial theory binds the theoretical to the personal in ways that are not straightforward or obvious. As I wrote, I was constantly reminded of my own complicated relationship to my mother and, more than once, considered abandoning the project. I express my thanks and gratitude to those who enabled me to undertake this comparative study of Ettingerian psychoanalysis and Lacanian psychoanalysis and see it through to completion.

The origins of this book date back to the annual meeting of the American Psychoanalytic Association meeting in Washington in 2011. At the conference, I met Dr. Angelina Rodriguez who was, at that time, teaching at the Universidad de Guanajuato, Mexico. Over dinner with a group of psychoanalytic scholars, Angelina introduced me to the theories of Bracha L. Ettinger. That evening in Washington was the beginning of a collegial exchange lasting many years. During that time, we read and spoke about Ettingerian psychoanalysis and art. The long-distance correspondence led to a decision to invite Bracha to exhibit her art-work in

Mexico and to present her work on the matrixial borderspace. She graciously accepted. Bracha met us in Toluca in 2014. We spent three weeks together traveling from Toluca, to Mexico City, to Guanajuato. Together, we spoke about the Feminine-matrixial, visited art galleries—including the Frida Kahlo Blue House—and genuinely got to know one another. Due to Angelina's incredible work with gallerists and curators in Mexico—I am an outsider to the Mexican art-scene—we organized two exhibitions of her work at the Galería Polivalente, Universidad de Guanajuato, Mexico; and the Museo Universitario Leopoldo Flores, Universidad Autónoma del Estado de México in Toluca.

I must also thank Bracha for being willing to fly from Israel to Mexico to meet us and to give lectures at the National Autonomous University of Mexico and at the Universidad de Gunajuato. Bracha devoted considerable time to presenting her scholarship on the matrixial and, in so doing, enabled me to better understand her critique of Lacan. Having made major contributions to theorizing the Feminine, ethics, and difference, it was a privilege to have concentrated time with Bracha. Viewing her paintings, notebooks, drawings, and video, in real time, added dimension and complexity to her writings on the Matrixial Borderspace. Bracha carried Indian inks and painted wherever we went. One of Bracha's Indian inks and aquarelle on paper appears on the cover of this book. It is titled Eurydice-Persephone (2021). (Without knowing it at the time, Bracha transmitted her passion for ink work to me and this is one of the things for which I am most grateful https://www.sheilacavanagh.ca/art.) Although the beauty, aesthetics, and sophistication of Bracha's art is beyond the scope of this book, it is, nevertheless, present in her theories of the Feminine-matrixial. Her visual art depicts mythological female figures, including, but not limited to, Eurydice, Medusa, Ophelia, and Persephone. The historical traumas of women, the mother in particular, during the German-Jewish Holocaust are witnessed in her work. Bracha's critical body of work, artistic and scholarly, is in dialogue with her familial legacy, including ancestor's imprisonment in the Stutthof Concentration Camp for Women during World War II.

During my sabbatical that year in Mexico, and later in Australia, I studied Bracha's writings and critiques of Lacanian psychoanalysis. I am grateful to York University for awarding me research sabbaticals, thus giving me much needed time to write; to the Social Sciences and Humanities Research Council of Canada (SSHRC) for supporting my scholarship through the Insight Grant SR ID 0548543 award; and to Varuna, the National Writers' House of Australia, where I wrote several chapters of this book. I would also like to thank Professor Alison M. Downham Moore of Western Sydney University for her friendship and for giving me a place to stay and write during not one, but two sabbaticals.

Before completing this book, I published several articles on Ettingerian psychoanalysis, Lacanian theory, and transgender studies in *Studies in Gender and Sexuality* (2022, 2019, and 2016); *Psychoanalysis, Culture & Society* (2022); *Transgender Studies Quarterly* (2018); *Sitegeist: A Journal for Psychoanalysis and Philosophy* (2018); *MAMSIE: Studies in the Maternal* (2017); and *European Journal of Psychoanalysis* (2016). I am exceedingly grateful to the anonymous reviewers and to the editors of all these journals. Without their critical feedback and insight, I would not have been able to develop my comparative analysis of Bracha's work and Lacanian psychoanalysis as fully as I have done. Equally, I am grateful to Dr. Patricia Gherovici and Dr. Manya Steinkoler for publishing my chapter titled "Tiresias and the Other Sexual Difference: Jacques Lacan and Bracha L. Ettinger" in their book titled *Psychoanalysis, Gender and Sexuality: From Feminism to Trans** (Cambridge University Press) that one the Gradiva book award for best edited collection.

Psychoanalytic scholarship is dependent upon communities of scholars and clinicians who, often without institutional support, make space for analytic inquiry, discussion, and debate. I am indebted to an international community of Lacanian scholars in Canada and the United States who have, through their friendship, labor, and scholarship, built an intellectual environment where I could write my book. Specifically, I thank those affiliated with the Association of Psychoanalysis, Culture & Society (APCS), especially Dr. Michael Loughlin and Dr. Angie Voela who coedit the *Psychoanalysis, Culture & Society* journal in which Julian Gutierrez-Albilla and I edited a Special Issue on Ettingerian psychoanalysis (2022). I also thank my Lacanian colleagues on the LACK Central Committee—LACK is an organization devoted to the promotion and development of thought in the tradition of Lacanian psychoanalytic theory and German

Idealism which has bi-annual conferences. Committee members include Dr. Jennifer Friedlander, Dr. Henry Krips, Dr. Todd McGowan, and Dr. Hilary Neroni. Through these bi-annual conferences, I am always inspired and encouraged by my friends and colleagues who include: Dr. Clint Burnham, Dr. Jessica Datema, Dr. Jill Gentile, Dr. Patricia Gherovici, Dr. Derek Hook, Dr. Sheldon George, Dr. Gouffrant, Dr. Don Kunze, Dr. Carol Owens, Dr. Fredrika Stjärne, Dr. Manya Steinkoler, and Dr. Stephanie Swales. I was first introduced to Lacanian thought through the Speaking of Lacan series in Toronto run by Dr. Mavis Himes (founded by the late William Ernest Robinson (1930–2023). Later, I attended colloquia and seminars offered at Après-Coup in New York City, an association for the study and transmission of Lacanian psychoanalysis; and presentations given at Lacan Toronto, a working-group that promotes the study and practice of Lacanian psychoanalysis run by Dr. Judith Hamilton. My psychoanalytic colleagues in Toronto have also encouraged my study, and I give particular thanks to Dr. David Dorenbaum, Dr. Patricia Elliot, Dr. Oren Gozlan, Dr. Judith Hamilton, Dr. Mavis Himes, Dr. Ilan Kapoor, Dr. Clive Thompson, and Dr. Christopher Vanderwees.

In 2022, I began my formation as a Lacanian psychoanalyst at the Lacan School of Psychoanalysis in California, United States. In this community of psychoanalysts and scholars, I was given a platform to share and develop my work in Lacanian studies. Without their clinical and intellectual support, I could not imagine having completed this book. In particular, I thank Dr. Shanna Carlson de la Torre, Dr. Christopher Chamberlin, Dr. Diana Cuello, Courtney Douds, Marcelo Estrada, Dr. Cécile Gouffrant, Dr. Christopher Meyer, Dr. Annie Rogers, Dr. Stephanie Swales, and Dr. Christopher Vanderwees.

Over the last decade, I hired two incredible doctoral research assistants, Caitlen Jensen and Hannah Maitland. Both have done incredible work editing, formatting, and preparing the text for publication. Following my proposal submission to Palgrave, I received two generous and entirely affirming reviews. I truly hope these reviewers will read this acknowledgment and know how much their endorsement means to me. I was delighted when the prolific scholar-analyst Dr. Jamieson Webster agreed to write the Foreword to my book. Given her insight into Bracha's art combined with her knowledge of Lacanian psychoanalysis, Jamieson is especially well-positioned to provide a scholarly context by way of introduction.

Last but not least, I thank Dr. Calum Neill and Dr. Derek Hook who edit the Palgrave Lacan Book Series. Both have done incredible work developing the Lacanian field and supporting a new generation of Lacanian scholars.

Competing Interests The author has no competing interests to declare that are relevant to the content of this manuscript.

Contents

1

Introduction

Bracha L. Ettinger is an internationally acclaimed artist,[1] feminist theorist, philosopher, and psychoanalyst whose scholarship makes important contributions to psychoanalytic theory. She contends that psychoanalytic theory, Lacanian theory more specifically, neglects the Feminine dimension of experience. In her theorization, the Feminine involves the m/Other, procreation, and the Woman (as distinct from female gender identity). Her critique spans from Freud to Lacan and is largely concerned with the over emphasis upon Oedipal sexual difference in Freud and the central importance of the phallus (as signifier) in Lacan. There is a concordant lack of emphasis upon what she calls the Other axis of

[1] Ettinger's art work has received international acclaim and she is at the vanguard of New European Painting. She has had solo exhibitions at Freud's Dream Museum in St. Petersburg (2013); The State Museum of the History of St. Petersburg (2013); Casco, Utrecht (2012); Musée des Beaux-Arts d'Angers, France (2011); Fundació Antoni Tàpies, Barcelona (2010); Kuvataideakatemia, Helsinki (2009); Freud Museum, London (2009); Gerwood Gallery, Oxford (2003); La librairie, Les Abattoirs, Toulouse (2003); Maison de France, Jerusalem (2002); the Drawing Center in New York City (2001); Pori Art Museum, Finland (1996); the Israel Museum (1995); the Pompidou Centre (1987, 1996, 2010–2011); the Museum of Calais (1988); and a Retrospective at the Centre for Fine Arts (The Palais des Beaux Arts) (2000) in Brussels. Feminist art historian Griselda Pollock has written about Ettinger's art in *Encounters in the Virtual Feminist Museum* as have another of others.

S. L. Cavanagh, *Bracha L. Ettinger and Jacques Lacan*, The Palgrave Lacan Series,
https://doi.org/10.1007/978-3-032-23293-9_1

sexual difference involving the Woman, which is, as we will see in later chapters, a complex borderlinking between partial-subjects. To the extent that the Feminine is theorized in the Freudian and Lacanian field, it is subsumed into either the Oedipal model (Freud) or the phallic model (Lacan). Ettinger explains that Freud's work on psychosexual development takes the male-masculine subject as the point of reference, while the female-feminine subject is anomalous. Oedipal sexuality is assumed to be neutral and universal. Even Lacan, who interprets the phallus as a signifier of lack (as opposed to an organ), is, in Ettinger's view, "not neutral but male" (2006d, 61). In her analysis, both Oedipal sex difference and phallic logic are specific to the "male body, to its pleasures and pains and to the phantasies attached to it" (2006d, 179). While Freud and Lacan knew that everyone can be Oedipal and phallic regardless of sexual morphology, Ettinger's theoretical wager is that there is something relating to the Feminine inclusive of reproductive capacity that warrants a critical feminist revision of Lacanian psychoanalysis.

In this book, I situate Ettinger's theory of the matrixial in Lacanian psychoanalysis so that we can more fully appreciate her critical feminist intervention and supplement, but also to consider those elements in the Lacanian corpus that involve the Feminine dimension of experience inclusive of matrixial subjectivity. Ettinger's critical supplement is one of the most elaborate feminist reinterpretations of Lacanian terms and concepts relating to the Feminine and the m/Other published to date. As such, the Lacanian origins and points of departure, relating to the matrixial, cannot be sidelined.

Given the central importance of the Feminine in Ettingerian theory, feminist scholars in a wide range of disciplines have eagerly engaged her theorization of the matrixial borderspace and published important works in a wide range of disciplines (Baraitser 2013; Cejudo-Escamilla 2021; Daly 2021; Kinsella 2019; Kisiel 2017, 2019, 2020, 2022; MacNamara 2021, 2024; Rodriguez 2016; Sander 2024; Simon 2024; Solstreif-Pirker 2022, 2023, and Wierzchowska 2022). It should not be surprising that feminist scholars, including those who read psychoanalysis, engage Ettinger's work on the matrixial (as noted above). What is surprising, however, is the lack of engagement on the part of Lacanian scholars. While there are notable exceptions (Malone 1997; Voela 2014; Voela and

Esin 2021; and Neill 2008), the lacuna of Lacanian writing on Ettinger's work is disappointing. It may also speak to an unwillingness on the part of Lacanians to engage feminist psychoanalytic thought. As noted above, the matrixial borderspace is developed in conversation with Lacanian psychoanalysis. By engaging feminist critiques and supplemental readings of Lacan, we may better understand the nuances, limitations, and possibilities of his teachings. Although Ettinger's writings are vast and differentiated in scope, this book focuses on those aspects of Ettingerian theory that engage, are relevant to, and critique Lacan's ideas regarding Feminine sexuality and the m/Other.

Unlike other feminist psychoanalytic scholars writing in the French tradition, like, for instance, Julia Kristeva, Luce Irigaray, and Hélène Cixous, Ettinger is less well known. But, her impressive body of scholarship is, increasingly, being featured in psychoanalytic circles. Indeed, her writings on the girl-daughter and the mother are much needed additions to the psychoanalytic literature. Ettinger's work on the matrixial and in what she calls the Other Sexual Difference (OSD) gives us a way to reconsider psychic struggles specific to the girl-daughter and possible future mother. Although the matrixial is not intended to be gendered or of relevance only to cisgender female-bodied people, it takes the Real, Imaginary, and Symbolic coordinates of female sexual morphology into account, especially as related to reproductive capacity. As I have argued in my own scholarship, Ettinger's writing on the Feminine is relevant to transgender studies and should not be interpreted in cisgender or essentialist terms (Cavanagh 2016a, 2018, 2019, 2022a, and 2022b). In fact, Ettinger wrote an article titled "Transgressing With-In-To the Feminine" (2000) that calls Lacan to task for saying that the man can know nothing of the Feminine dimension of experience.

In fact both Lacan and Ettinger refer to the mythical character Tiresias,[2] appearing in the Oedipal trilogy, a pivotal and understudied figure in psychoanalysis who changes sex. In 1960, at the University of Amsterdam, Lacan delivered a paper later published in *Écrits* (Ettinger 2006d), saying

[2]Tiresias appears in Homer's *Odyssey* and has an important role in Sophocles' tragedies *Antigone*, *Oedipus the King*, and in *Oedipus at Colonus* as well as in Euripides' *Phoenician Women*, among other literary and theatrical works. Tiresias reappears in high modernism in T.S. Eliot's "The Waste Land".

we should not be fooled by Tiresias; the mythological character cannot know anything more about Feminine sexuality than we do, which amounts to nothing. For Lacan, the Feminine is a mystery out of symbolic bounds. But for Ettinger, the Feminine is relevant to everyone regardless of gender identity or sexual positioning. She writes: "Under the matrixial light, the transgression in the figure of Tiresias between man and woman is not a transgression of a frontier between known maleness and unknown femaleness". Rather, since the "matrixial *I* carries traces of experiences of the matrixial *non-I*, inasmuch as I know in the other and my other knows in me, non-knowledge of the feminine, in the matrixial borderspace, is impossible, by virtue of the transgression itself" (Ettinger 2000, 189, emphasis in original).

In my reading, Ettingerian theories relating to the Feminine provide a way to understand the importance of transgender subjectivity and of interpreting sexuality beyond cisgender binaries. But what I foreground in this book is the way Ettingerian psychoanalysis sheds light on the unique predicaments of girl-daughters who, perhaps like transfeminine people in some ways, struggle to become women. By focusing on the case study of Dora, *The Ravishing of Lol Stein* by Marguerite Duras and *Antigone* of the Oedipal trilogy, I demonstrate the originality of the Ettingerian analysis without losing track of the ways her theorization is indebted to Lacan. Indeed, I show how both theorists must be read together.

Despite a growing interest in Ettingerian scholarship, some non-psychoanalytic feminist scholars who read Ettingerian theory lack a nuanced understanding of Lacanian concepts, theories, and ideas relating to sexuation, the m/Other, the signifier, *object a*, and the unconscious. As a result, Lacanian theory is often dismissed as phallocentric and the central importance of Lacanian formulations to Ettingerian theory are misunderstood, de-emphasized, or neglected entirely.[3] In some instances, there is an earnest attempt to situate Ettinger in Lacanian thought by feminists less familiar with Lacan but, too often, they take Ettinger's cri-

[3] Anna Louise Johnson (2006) claimed in her doctoral dissertation that an exclusive examination of Ettinger and Lacan "inhibits an understanding of the nature of Ettinger's Lacanianism" (8) and that an "adequate assessment of the general validity and significance of the theory of the matrix is occluded by a confrontation with Lacanian psychoanalysis" (8).

tique of Lacan at face value; thereby reproducing Ettinger's critique of Lacan without the benefit of having read and studied Lacan (Smith 2013).[4] While Ettinger critiques Lacan, she does not recommend a wholesale dismissal of Lacanian ideas relating to phallic sexuality. In fact, she calls herself a feminist post-Lacanian theorist. Ettinger's position is that Lacanian theory is limited to the extent that it does not sufficiently engage the Feminine dimension of experience relating to reproduction and the m/Other.

While Lacan viewed the Feminine as out of Symbolic bounds (akin to a void or eclipse), the Feminine-matrixial, in Ettingerian theory, is felt and non-consciously known through aesthetic and affective fields. This supplementary dimension occurs alongside but is not delimited by the Lacanian Symbolic. For Ettinger, the Lacanian Symbolic deals with "whole objects, one-ness, sameness, all-ness, and symmetry" (Ettinger 1992, 193). The matrixial-Feminine is not about castrating cuts, splits, and signifiers. The matrixial borderspace is about borderlinking as I explain more fully in the following chapter. It is a sub-Symbolic where we exist, as partial-subjects, in relation to Others (as *non-I*'s). Building upon Lévinas, Ettinger contends that the Feminine is about the future, ethics, and the trans-subjective (whereby we are more than One).

In their discussion of Ettinger's feminist thought and mythology, Vanda Zaijko and Miriam Leonard (2006) explain that the Feminine is an "inter/trans-subjectivizing structure/encounter/space where potentially human subjects co-emerge and co-transform" (30). This is to say that the Ettingerian subject is an encounter-event which she likens to a condition of transitivity. For Ettinger, otherness exists within the subject and we are borderlinked to our partners-in-difference in shared matrixial webs. What is crucial to understand is that the Feminine-matrixial challenges the belief in what Ettinger calls "subjectivity supported by a One (separate or fused)" (2006d, 87).

While object relations theory informs Ettinger's analytic of the matrixial, her notion of the Feminine is not about relationality. Relationality involves whole (castrated) subjects. The Ettingerian Feminine is a

[4] Notable exceptions include Kareen Ror Malone (1997) and Angie Voela (2014), and Voela and Esin (2021).

non-conscious borderspace whereby we are interlinked as partial-subjects. This iteration of the Feminine is predicated upon a "borderline coming-into-being" (Ettinger 2007, 119). What comes into being is the Woman who, in the Ettingerian model, exists, but not as subject. The Woman is the "co-emerging partial self and Other, or a different kind of relations to the Other" (Bracha Lichtenberg Ettinger 2006d, 72). The Ettingerian Woman involves "different conditions of subjective co-emergence[s]" (Pollock 2006, 31) in a Feminine-matrixial field that is composed of the "I with/for *some* other(s)" (Bracha Lichtenberg Ettinger 2006d, 116). As I will explain more fully in Chap. 3, Ettinger's Woman is the Other of the masculine/feminine opposition.

While the Lacanian Woman also does not exist in phallic terms, it is, paradoxically, her non-existence that gives her an exceptional status. She is, unlike the man, not-all subordinated to the phallic premise. But for Ettinger, Lacan's notion of the Woman is limited to the extent that it is developed in phallic terms, thereby obfuscating the Feminine dimension. As a result, Lacan's writing on Feminine sexuality is, for Ettinger, "articulated via the model of male 'castration' and paternal prohibition or is equated with pure bodily experience, whereas the phallus is considered as the only 'signifier of signifiers' for sexual difference" (1997, 367). The Woman is not-all there, an object of exchange, or, in Ettinger's common refrain, reduced to an "inaccessible Other/Thing/*object a* as absence" (1997, 367) in the Lacanian field. This is what leads Ettinger to conclude that we are "trapped in the language of the phallus" (11) and that Freudian and Lacanian psychoanalysis are phallocentric.

For Ettinger, the Woman is not best understood as a hole in the Real or as the Thing (*das Ding*) which originates with the m/Other in the Lacanian paradigm. The Woman is something more than *object a* (cause of man's desire). In the Ettingerian definition, Woman is not a subject per se, but a condition of transitivity. While transitivity is usually thought to be regressive and infantile, it is, for Ettinger, central to the OSD in the matrixial borderspace. Moreover, matrixial transitivity is subjectifying and relevant to the clinic of psychoanalysis. From the perspective of the matrixial, Woman is a "border-Other, a becoming in-ter-with the Other, never a radical alterity" (Ettinger 2001, 129). There is no one isolated subject in Ettinger's formulation of the matrixial, only partial-subjects bound to Others (or *non-I*'s) in a matrixial web.

The British art historian Griselda Pollock is the most prolific feminist scholar interpreting Ettinger's work (1994, 1996, 1999, 2004, 2005, 2007, 2009a, 2009b, 2014, 2016, 2017, 2019; Pollock, Griselda 2013) and speculates that matrixial-Feminine desire might "signify something of profound importance for discussions of human subjectivity and indeed sociality" (2006d, 22). Pollock published the first English-language introduction to Ettingerian psychoanalysis in *Differences: a journal of feminist cultural studies* (1992). Her works on Ettinger focus on art theory, feminist ethics, the maternal, trauma, aesthetics, representation, and the Feminine. While Pollock's contribution to interpreting and promulgating Ettingerian psychoanalysis is important and unparalleled in scope, it is largely critical of Lacanian psychoanalysis. Although she acknowledges the Lacanian antecedents in Ettinger's writings, Pollock seems to regard Lacan as being phallocentric as opposed to interpreting the structure of phallocentrism. I maintain that there is a critical difference between analyzing the phallic signifier (which lacks) and endorsing it. Pollock is largely responsible for bringing Ettingerian art and scholarship to an international audience, but she does not, unfortunately, engage Lacanian feminist writings that seek to interpret the phallic signifier as relating to the Real (unrepresentable) structure of sexual difference. For Pollock, as for Ettinger, Lacan is phallocentric and, although both scholars know that the phallus is not equivalent to the penis-organ, the metonymy is tied to male anatomy and cannot be used to designate the Feminine dimension. But more than this, the phallic structure Lacan theorizes is not neutral but articulated from a masculine-phallic point of view. This is a legitimate and important critique that I explore throughout this book. But I question two underlying premises: one, that the phallus essentially belongs to, or must be attributed to the penis-organ (and to men more broadly); and two, that the phallic structure does not itself include aspects of the Feminine elaborated upon by Ettinger.

As Lacanian readers will be quick to note, there is no shortage of phallic women in Lacanian teachings and that the phallus comes up lacking. It is a signifier with no essential meaning. The phallus is an Imaginary object (*ab-sens*) that Lacan theorizes in relation to the Real and to the

Symbolic. It does not exist as such, but it has a function. Feminist scholars who specialize in Lacanian psychoanalysis, including Joan Copjec (2002, 2004, 2015. 2018), Juliet Mitchell and Jacqueline Rose (1983); Ellie Ragland (2008, 2012, 2014), Jacqueline Rose (2005), Kaja Silverman (1992); Collette Soler (2002a, 2002b, 2006, 2012, 2023), Alenka Zupančič (2017) and many others, make the case that the phallus is not an organ, but a third term that stands in for difference itself. It could be argued that the phallus enables the Feminine because it marks an absent-exceptional space. Moreover, as a third term, the phallus cannot be masculine *or* feminine. It is the unrepresentable difference between the two. In Lacanian terms, the phallus signifies a lack in the Other and, thus, becomes a signifier of the desire of the Other. This phallus concerns sexuality, but is not a thing-object-organ that can be had or obtained. Nor is it meant to legitimize a male-masculine socio-cultural order whereby women lack in a negative way.

In my review of the feminist literature on Ettingerian psychoanalysis, Kareen Ror Malone (1997) is the only one to question Ettinger's claim regarding a phallic bias in Lacan. Building upon Lacanian feminist interpretations, Malone (1997) explains that the Lacanian phallus gives us access (however partial and flawed) to the desire of the m/Other. More significantly, this access needs to be interpreted alongside the Ettingerian matrixial which, for Malone (1997), is not (only) about the Feminine, but the non-part of the Symbolic Order that is the "other/outside place" (420) and culturally marginalized.

I do not focus on Lacanian antecedents to detract from Ettinger's original interventions. Rather, I seek to situate Ettingerian psychoanalysis in Lacanian theory. This book focuses on Ettinger's critical supplement to Lacanian theory vis-a-vis the Feminine. I draw attention to the segments of Lacanian theorizing relevant to the Feminine and the m/Other so that we can better understand and evaluate the matrixial supplement alongside Ettinger's critical intervention. By reading Ettinger in relation to Lacan, we may better understand critical differences and areas of contiguity in their respective theorizing.

To read Ettinger and Lacan together, feminist scholars must be open to questioning long held presumptions about Lacanian phallocentrism. Equally, Lacanians must read feminist psychoanalytic theory and commit to inquiries relating to the eclipse of the Feminine and its consequences. If feminists read Lacan through the lens of biology, or through a structural logic that does not take (phallic) lack into account (de la Torre 2018), we miss something vital in the synergy between Ettinger and Lacan. My contention is that Ettinger must be read and interpreted in relation to Lacan. Not only does Ettingerian psychoanalysis emerge as a critical response to Lacanian psychoanalysis, but the discourse of the matrixial is based on terminology deriving from the Lacanian lexicon. In fact, the "matrix" derives from Lacan's 1938 essay titled "Familial Complexes in the Formation of the Individual." In his early work, Lacan used the term matrix to denote not only the mother, but the "*sevrage*" from the mother that occurs during weaning. To be precise, Lacan writes that a "primordial weaning…separates the infant at birth from its matrix" (31/15, Quoted in Barzilai 1999).

It is difficult to think about the Real of procreation in Lacanian terms unless, of course, we return to his early writings on the "weaning complex" (Barzilai 1999), which, unfortunately, contemporary Lacanians tend to ignore in their prioritization of his later works. While several authors engage the question of the maternal and the m/Other in Lacanian theory, only Barzilai (1999) and Smart (2021) do so with studied expertise in Lacanian theory (1999, 2021). Apart from these two exceptional works, few Lacanians interested in the question of the Feminine have built upon Lacan's early references to the problem of *sevrage* from the mother's body (Barzilai 1999); what Lacan calls the law of the mother (Smart 2021); *la langue* (the mother tongue) (Cixous 2009; J. Kristeva 1973, 1980); the way Freudian notions of castration are reconfigured, in Lacan, to date back to weaning [*sevrage*] (as opposed to the Oedipal Complex); the "anxiety [l'angoisse] born with life" (quoted in Barzilai 1999, 30); Lacan's engagement with Melanie Klein's writing on the mother (Borossa et al., 2015); and Otto Rank's thesis on the trauma of birth (2015). As a result, the relevance of the m/Other and the Feminine more generally to Lacanian psychoanalysis have been neglected. As a result, vital elements of Lacanian theory relating to the Feminine, the m/Other, procreation and weaning are ignored or, at least, sidelined.

Ettinger's work enables a return to Lacan, but through new feminist formulations of the m/Other, the Woman, and the matrix. As I will discuss more fully in the following chapter, the matrix is intended to represent a heterogeneous Feminine difference. Much like the Lacanian phallus is not intended to represent the penis but is, nevertheless gendered, the matrix is not intended to represent the womb but is also, unfortunately, gendered. For Ettinger, the matrix is an "unconscious borderspace" that remembers female bodily specificity but is not based on "essence, identity, or negation" (1997, 368). While it is difficult to think outside bigendered grids, the matrixial is best understood as non-sex-specific borderlinkings. Ettinger writes:

> The matrixial difference emerges...*beyond* the binary difference between the sexes – whether it is understood biologically (male/female) or in terms of identities (masculine/feminine). This archaic minimal difference before and beside repression and castration points to different kinds of "holes" in the Real, and to the difference of their traces. (2006, 56)

The beyond of binary sex difference enables us to theorize not only matrixial traces in the borderlinking but also a return to Lacanian ideas about the mother-matrix. Ettinger elaborates upon the sphere of the matrix, and the Feminine more generally, that is underdeveloped in Lacan. Specifically, she invites a return to Lacan's writings on the trace of the signifier, but also to the *object a* as a trace enabled by lack, as opposed to an object lost.

In Pollock's astute assessment of Ettingerian psychoanalysis, she considers how it opens up a new avenue in feminist psychoanalytic theorizing relating to subjectivity. The matrix "allows into discourse a stratum of human subjectivization framed by the invisible specificity of the female body" (Pollock 2001, 118). From a Lacanian standpoint, this involves the Real of the body. But the question of how to theorize being in relation to the Real of the female-reproductive body is one Lacan did not answer, at least not to Ettinger's satisfaction. For her, this question requires a new model of subjectivization. Ettinger posits a formulation of sub-subjectivity that involves multiplicity, severality, and elements of the Feminine, grounded not only in conception and scenes of birth, but maternality. While severality (the subject-with-others) is developed in relation to the Lacanian notion of *sevrage*, Ettingerian psychoanalysis is about links as opposed to cuts: borderlinkings as opposed to castrating cuts. These matrixial borderlinkages are central to subjectivity. But most importantly, for Ettinger, they derive from the m/Other and give rise to an Other (non-phallic) axis of sexual difference.

The Other Sexual Difference

The OSD is Ettinger's answer to Oedipal/phallic sexual difference (Freud and Lacan respectively). It is closely related to Lacan's later work on Feminine sexuality, inclusive of the Real, the m/Other, jouissance, and the sinthôme. But the OSD is not reducible to the Oedipal Complex. Nor is it mediated by the phallic signifier. Before sexual difference in phallic terms becomes thinkable, the subject's difference from the mother (as first Other) is paramount. The OSD is based on the late prenatal period, whereby the subject-to-be and the mother-to-be are co-relating but not characterized by fusion, symbiosis, or psychosis. The first axis of sexual difference is a difference the child must negotiate with and from the m/Other. The first order of sexual difference does not involve the other sex, but the difference of the becoming-subject from the m/Other. The OSD continues to emerge before, during, and after Oedipalization but is not delimited by the psychosexual developmental stages narrated by Freud. Nor is it arbitrated by the phallic signifier. In fact, the OSD pre-dates the signifier, which structures what are, for Lacan, two ways of being: masculine or Feminine in relation to the Other's lack. The OSD apprehends "differences in the linking in-between *I* and *non-I* – not a difference (same or opposite) *from* the *non-I*" (Ettinger 2004, 89). The first *non-I* is the mother-to-be experienced by the subject-to-be through joint sensations and affective links in utero.

For Ettinger the OSD is not about sexuation in Lacanian terms. Sexuation is about castrated subjects, whereas the OSD involves severality. Severality refers to an aggregated subjectivity whereby the *I* (as partial-subject) exists in relation to their *non-I*s (Others, partners in difference). The Ettingerian subject-as-several is transitive. But matrixial transitivity is subjectifying, not infantile or regressive. It is about non-conscious borderlinkings to Others that can be felt and intuited but not signified in

Lacanian terms. The OSD involves an element of being, in relation to the Feminine, that "struggles to open up, a difference that has nothing to do with Oedipal man/woman difference, but which accompanies and subtends it" (Bracha Lichtenberg Ettinger 2006d, 89). These elements of being are not reducible to the Other jouissance theorized by Lacan. But the OSD does involve desire and Eros. "Matrixial desire is an aspiration and an inspiration from a feminine *jouissance* toward the edges of a wider Symbolic" (113).

Ettinger calls the wider Symbolic a matrixial sub-Symbolic. From a Lacanian perspective, this sub-stratum is Real (beyond language and sight). But it can, from an Ettingerian perspective, be apprehended through a matrixial gaze (a modification of the phallic gaze theorized by Lacan) as we shall see in a later chapter. The matrixial gaze is an affective-touching gaze; it is fuzzy and intercepts borderline differences best characterized as linkages (as opposed to cuts). To put this in another way, the matrix enables "early recognition of invisible difference" (Ettinger 1992, 193) and is, for Ettinger, a sub-Stratum where (and when) elements of the Feminine are felt-sensed. Not only does the Feminine-matrixial tap into an otherness that is Feminine, but also it is a grounding for ethics: an ethics that involves "unknown others" (Ettinger 1992, 12).

Bracha Litchenberg Ettinger

Bracha L. Ettinger was born in Mandatory Palestine in 1948 but spent many years in Paris, France. She did her analytic formation in Paris with senior analysts influenced by Jacques Lacan, including Piera Auglanier (1923–1990), Françoise Dolto, Pierre Fédida (1934–2002), Nicolas Abraham (1919–1975), Mária Török (1925–1998), and Jacques-Alain Miller. Prior to that, she trained at the London Centre for Psychotherapy, the Tavistock Clinic, and at the Philadelphia Association. She was a professor at the European Graduate School in Switzerland and at The Global Centre for Advanced Studies in Dublin, Ireland, while maintaining both a clinical and art practice. Ettinger has also held visiting and research professorships at the University of Leeds and elsewhere. Having been born to Jewish-Polish Holocaust survivors, Ettinger's artistic and scholarly works engage and respond to modern atrocities in Europe and the Middle East: the Shoah and the Nakba in particular. Much of Ettinger's early art-work contains references to psychiatric diagnosis of female ailments,[5] images of Jews in concentration camps and of her extended family, some of whom were imprisonment in the Stutthof Concentration Camp for Women during World War II. Her art-works center upon Jewish women and mothers during the Nazi-German Holocaust, along with elements of memory, trauma, discordance of time, and the Feminine.[6]

Ettinger's scholarship and art broach a wide range of topics relating to feminist ethics, philosophy, psychoanalysis, art, literature, aesthetics, exile, borders, time, memory, and mythology. The most enduring mythological figures in her scholarly and artistic works combined include Antigone, Jocasta, Diotima, Persephone, and Eurydice.[7] Through these figures, Ettinger elaborates upon inter-generational trauma and the importance of what she calls *wit(h)nessing* (a matrixial variation on witnessing) in and through a matrixial stratum of difference. Together, her theory and artwork forms a matrixial covenant upon which Ettinger develops a feminist psychoanalytic theory of otherness, the Feminine, and the matrixial with attention to procreation. Through her art and academic production, Ettinger alters and develops upon Lacan's formative work on sexuation—particularly as it relates to the Woman and to what he calls the non-existent sexual relation.

Ettinger began to publish her writings on the matrixial borderspace in the 1990s. The corpus of her theory is inspired by the work of Wilfred Bion, Sigmund Freud, Emmanual Levinas, Maurice Merleau-Ponty, Gilles Deleuze and Félix Guattari, Donald Winnicot, and, as already

[5] Bracha L. Ettinger, Matrix – Family Album, n.7, 200302005. Mixed media and oil Painting.

[6] I write this book as Palestine faces genocidal actions by the Israeli government and polarization between Israeli and Palestinian artists escalates in European arts and cultural institutions. For a reference to Ettinger's decision to withdraw from Documenta, an exhibition of European contemporary art whose shareholders "do not tolerate Finding Committee members having BDS [Boycott, Divestment, Sanctions] affiliations, See: Lentchner (2023) and Greenberger (2023).

[7] Eurydice is the subject of Ettinger's art series 'From Eurydice---Pieta series, 2013–2020' that has been shown internationally. Eurydice, the figure of Greek mythology, who disappears under the gaze of her lover, Orpheus, is also used in Ettinger's scholarly work to differentiate the matrixial gaze from the Lacanian (phallic) gaze.

discussed, Lacan. Ettinger's first main English publication on the matrixial was in *Differences: a journal of feminist cultural studies*. The "Matrix and Metramorphosis" (Ettinger 1992) was followed by a series of additional articles and book chapters on different elements of the matrixial including, but not limited to, matrixial borderlines and borderlinkages (Ettinger 1994, 1996), the matrixial gaze (2001), matrixial trans-subjectivity (2006), the girl-to-m/other matrixial feminine difference (2006), matrixial aesthetics (2004), the matrixial Feminine (2017), etc. In 1993, Griselda Pollock published a lecture delivered by Ettinger in Leeds as a book which was reprinted in *The Matrixial Borderspace* (2006d). This is the first and most often cited book collection featuring original writings by Ettinger (edited by Massumi 2006). In *The Matrixial Borderspace*, Masumi showcases Ettinger's most important works relating to the Feminine matrixial.

But before this inaugural book, Ettingerian theory was featured in a special issue of *Theory, Culture & Society* (2004) edited by Roy Boyne. The issue contains articles on Ettingerian psychoanalysis by Judith Butler, Griselda Pollock, Roy Boyne, Jean-François Lyotard, Lone Bertelsen, Couze Venn, Sophie Arkette, and Ettinger herself. The writings focus on the Ettingerian notion of the Other, her art-work inspired by Eurydice, Feminine aesthetics relating to the matrixial, memory, amamnesis, and the visible.

Some of the most esteemed scholars engaging Ettingerian psychoanalysis include Griselda Pollock as already mentioned, Judith Butler, Catherine de Zegher, Jean-François Lyotard, Christine Buci-Glucksmann, and Brian Massumi. Ettinger's theories of the matrixial, along with her paintings and art notebooks, have also been written about by psychoanalysts of distinct paradigms and orientations (Baraitser et al. 2010; Giffney et al. 2009; Rowley 1999; Walsh 2011). Not surprisingly, much has been written on Ettingerian art, theory, and matrixial aesthetics (Bourriaud 2014; Fisher 2024; Kisiel 2017, 2020; Van Loo 2009; Vigneault 2011). Julián Daniel Gutiérrez-Albilla (2022) has used Ettinger's formulation of the matrixial to theorize the cinema of Pedro Almodóvar. I have published a body of work that applies Ettingerian psychoanalysis to transgender studies (Cavanagh 2016a, 2016b, 2018, 2019, 2019a, 2019b, 2022, 2022a, and 2022b). More recently, Albilla and I co-edited a special issue of *Psychoanalysis, Culture & Society* (2022) on Ettingerian psychoanalysis with a Foreword by Griselda Pollock. This special issue features a range of works on art, television, organ transplants, environmental ethics, and transgender studies.

Since the early 2000s, Ettinger's scholarship has been widely cited and is making immeasurable contributions to feminist psychoanalytic thought; contributions that can be compared to those made by Julia Kristeva, Luce Irigaray, and Hélène Cixous. It is clear that Ettingerian psychoanalysis has influenced a wide range of subject-areas, but this book is confined to those elements of the matrixial borderspace most relevant to Lacanian psychoanalysis. More specifically, I put Ettinger into conversation with Lacan to better understand the contribution and challenge her theory of the matrixial borderspace offers to Lacanian teachings about Feminine sexuality, the Other jouissance, *object a* (*das Ding*), the gaze, and the m/Other.

Chapter Breakdown

Matrixial Borderspace

Chapter 2 introduces Ettinger's theory of the matrixial borderspace with attention to her critique of Freudian and Lacanian psychoanalysis. I focus on four central elements of matrixial theory relating to the Feminine: matrixial subjectivity; *metra*morphosis; matrixial gaze; and the borderlinking. I contextualize Ettinger's work in Freudian and Lacanian theory, but also in relation to Luce Irigaray and Julia Kristeva. Like Ettinger, Irigaray and Kristeva have developed critiques of Lacan from the vantage point of the Feminine. What distinguishes Ettinger from Irigaray and Kristeva, however, is the attention she gives to the subjectifying experience of pregnancy and to the matrixial sub-stratum. The matrixial dimension invites co-emergence and re-cognizes the Other—not as object (or *object a* in Lacanian terms)—but as extension of the subject *in* and *as* encounter. I show how the matrixial borderspace is not only inspired by a critique of Lacanian psychoanalysis but also a wish to illuminate a Feminine stratum of difference in Lacanian psychoanalysis.

The Other Sexual Difference

Chapter 3 outlines Bracha Ettinger's theory of the Other (Feminine) Sexual Difference with attention to her critique of Freud and Lacan. She contends that both neglect the relevance of procreation, pre-natal experience, and the m/Other in their respective theories. As a result, the matrixial dimensions of experience originating with the m/Other are submerged in Freud and Lacan. Moreover, the distinction between *being* and *having* of relevance to Lacan's understanding of sexual positioning cannot account for pregnancy and the way it occurs without psychotic fusion. Ettinger develops a theory of the OSD to supplement the Oedipal-phallic axis of unconscious sexuality which is, in her critical reflection, authored from the man's side. For Ettinger, the OSD is a Feminine sexual difference that originates with the m/Other. It is set in motion during the late prenatal period where the subject-to-be and the mother-to-be are borderlinked in utero. I show how Ettinger's theory of the matrixial-Feminine relates to the Lacanian formulation of the Feminine not-all and the Other.

The Ettingerian Woman

In Chap. 4, I discuss the Ettingerian definition of Woman and distinguish it from the Lacanian formulation of the Woman who does not exist. For Ettinger, Woman is a condition of transitivity that can be apprehended. She also refers to Woman as a "co-emerging partial self and Other, or a different kind of relations to the Other" (2006d, 72). I consider a relation between the Ettingerian Woman and the Lacanian notion of the Other. My contention is that matrixial transitivity bears a resemblance to Lacan's conceptualization of the Other and the intra-said [*intra-dit*]. Indeed, Lacan writes about elements of subjectivity relating to what he calls "inter-human relations" in his seminar on the psychosis. The problem, as Ettinger sees it, is that whenever Lacan speaks about the intra-said or the inter-human, he does so in relation to psychosis. Thus, putting the Feminine in close proximity to the psychotic. Ettinger's feminist supplement enables us to better understand the Feminine dimension of being along with what it means to have a relation to the Other in non-psychotic terms.

Following these three chapters on Ettingerian theory, I devote the next three chapters to fictional and real clinical cases interpreted by both scholar-analysts: Dora, Lol Stein, and Antigone. In these chapters, I consider the plight of the girl-daughter as understood by Ettinger and Lacan to illustrate difference and overlap in their respective approaches.

Dora: Hysteria and the Other Sexual Difference

This chapter illustrates the interpretations of the Freudian case study of Dora made by Bracha Ettinger and Jacques Lacan. Both critique Freud for neglecting the question of Dora's desire. For Lacan, Dora ponders what it means to be an object of desire and searches for a solution to the sexual non-rapport between the man and the Woman. For Ettinger, Dora grapples with the difference between the mother and the girl-becoming woman (Dora). Another point of distinction is in the way Lacan approaches the question of Dora's desire in relation to hysteria and the transference, whereas Ettinger argues that hysteria occurs when access to the Feminine dimension is blocked. For Ettinger, Dora needed to explore the enigma of femininity, what it means to desire and to be desired in/through/with an adult-woman in a matrixial alliance. While Lacan may neglect the matrixial sub-Stratum of relevance to Ettinger, I contend that he does engage what he calls another realm akin to the Ettingerian sub-Symbolic. Moreover, there is, in my reading, a correspondence between the Ettingerian notion of severality and Lacanian formulation of the Other.

Lol Stein: The Object, the Gaze, and the m/Other

Bracha Ettinger and Jacques Lacan wrote about the female protagonist in *The Ravishing of Lol Stein* by the late Marguerite Duras. Duras was a French feminist writer and luminary whose writing is best described as belonging to what Hélène Cixous defines as *Écriture feminine*. For Lacan, Duras reveals something vital about *object a* through the story of Lol Stein. In his view, Duras gives fictive form to the non-descript *Thing* animating desire, to the Woman (who, for him, does not exist), to the way we are ravished by the Other, subject to the gaze of the Other, occupy a void, and rendered naked before the Other. Ettinger foregrounds the m/Other and the other woman in her analysis of Lol Stein. In so doing, Ettinger revisits the Lacanian notion of the gaze and supplements it with the matrixial gaze; develops her conceptualization of the *a-link* as alternative to Lacan's *object a*; and articulates a matrixial version of the Lacanian *sinthôme*. Ettinger also develops what she calls the Jocasta Complex, a matrixial supplement to the Oedipal Complex. Her attention to the Feminine dimension of Lol Stein's symptomatology differs from Lacan's focus on the non-object of desire in the novel.

Antigone and the "Jocasta Complex"

Bracha Ettinger and Jacques Lacan agree that the Sophocles drama *Antigone* offers something significant to psychoanalytic ethics. Lacan is impressed by the way Antigone acts on her desire and takes leave from the Other symbolized by the King and his unjust law. Ettinger is impressed by the way Antigone is guided by a matrixial ethic that is un-signifiable in the polis. Although her radical act of burying Polynices (twice) puts her mortal life in danger, Antigone is, in Ettinger's interpretation, bound by a Feminine-matrixial ethic relating to life and futurity. Ettinger contends that the transgression is not about the second-death, the *Até*, beauty, and the limit as Lacan contends, but about the matrixial borderlinking whereby there is a supplementary value to the figure of the brother Polynices. Alongside the Ettingerian critique, I show how Lacan does not neglect the figure of the brother. I also contend that what Lacan refers to as beauty, radiating in the space between to two symbolically differentiated fields, is resonant with the matrixial sub-symbolic in Ettinger's theorization of the Feminine.

Ettinger and Lacan: A Sexual Impasse That Will Not Stop Being Written

The conclusion incorporates Lacan's writings on the m/Other, procreation, and the *Thing* (*das Ding*) more fully than in previous chapters to better understand the differences and points of overlap between Lacan and Ettinger. While some of Ettinger's writings posit Lacanian theory and matrixial theory as wholly distinct, there are, in fact, important areas of synergy and overlap that need to be acknowledged. Ettinger may be correct in her assessment of Freud's over-emphasis upon the Oedipal Complex and in her assessment of Lacan's foreclosure of the womb as a subjective space of difference, but there are, nevertheless, references to the womb and interpretations of the 'Weaning Complex' in Lacan's teachings that complicate Ettinger's assessment. My contention is that there are matrixial seeds planted in Lacan's work that Ettinger reformulates through her own feminist post-Lacanian discourse. But there is also a theoretical impasse between Lacan and Ettinger that concern sexual positioning, subjectivity, the m/Other and the Real.

Bibliography

Baraitser, Lisa. 2013. Collecting Time: Some Reflections on the Psychopolitics of Belonging. *New Formations* 79 (79): 8–25.

Baraitser, Lisa, Griselda Pollock, and Sigal Spigel. 2010. Editorial: M(O)Ther Trouble: Motherhood, Psychoanalysis, Feminism. *Studies in the Maternal* 2 (1): 1.

Barzilai, Shuli. 1999. *Lacan and the Matter of Origins. Lacan and the Matter of Origins.* Stanford, Calif: Stanford University Press.

Borossa, Julia, Catalina Bronstein, and Claire Pajaczkowska. 2015. The New Dialogues: Freud, Klein, Lacan. In *The New Klein-Lacan Dialogues*. United Kingdom: Taylor & Francis Group.

Bourriaud, Nicolas. 2014. Bracha Ettinger: Off (Hors) Figures. *Image & Text: A Journal for Design* 23 (1): 18–33.
Butler, Judith. 2006. Bracha's Eurydice. In *The Matrixial Borderspace*, Theory Out of Bounds, ed. Bracha Ettinger, vol. 28. Minneapolis: University of Minnesota Press.
Cavanagh, Sheila. 2016a. Tiresias and Psychoanalysis with/out Oedipus. *European Journal of Psychoanalysis* 28.
Cavanagh, Sheila L. 2016b. Transsexuality as Sinthome: Bracha L. Ettinger and the Other (Feminine) Sexual Difference. *Studies in Gender and Sexuality* 17 (1): 27–44. https://doi.org/10.1080/15240657.2016.1135681.
Cavanagh, Sheila. 2018. Bracha L. Ettinger, Jacques Lacan, and Tiresias: The Other Sexual Difference. *Sitegeist: A Journal for Psychoanalysis and Philosophy* 13:32–50.
Cavanagh, Sheila L. 2019. Transgender, Hysteria, and the Other Sexual Difference: An Ettingerian Approach. *Studies in Gender and Sexuality* 20 (1): 36–50. https://doi.org/10.1080/15240657.2019.1559517.
Cavanagh, Sheila L. 2019a. Tiresias: Bracha L. Ettinger and the Transgression with-in-to the Feminine. In *Femininity and Psychoanalysis*, ed. Agnieszka Piotrowska and Ben Tyrer, 1st ed., 204–216. United Kingdom: Routledge.
Cavanagh, Sheila L. 2019b. Transcryptums: An Ettingerian Reading of the Trans-Subjective Landscape in Transparent. *TSQ: Transgender Studies Quarterly* 6 (1): 20–42.
Cavanagh, Sheila. 2022. Tiresias and the Other Sexual Difference: Jacques Lacan and Bracha L. Ettinger. In *Psychoanalysis, Gender, and Sexualities: From Feminism to Trans*, ed. Patricia Gherovici and Manya Steinkoler, 197–211. Cambridge University Press.
Cavanagh, Sheila L. 2022a. The Matrixial Gaze: Transgender in Boys Don't Cry. *Studies in Gender and Sexuality* 23 (4): 243–255.
Cavanagh, Sheila L. 2022b. Transgender and the Other Sexual Difference in Vivek Shraya's Trisha. *Psychoanalysis, Culture & Society* 27 (4): 485–501.
Cavanagh, Sheila, and Julián Daniel Gutiérrez-Albilla, eds. (n.d.) 'Special Issue: "The Psychoanalysis of Bracha L. Ettinger"'. *Psychoanalysis, Culture & Society* 27 (4).
Cejudo-Escamilla, Sonia. 2021. Trauma and Transcryptum: Towards a Feminist Methodology for the Analysis of Narratives of Trauma. *Sociología y Tecnociencia* 11 (1): 104–124.
Cixous, Hélène. 2009. The Laugh of the Medusa. In *Feminisms Redux: An Anthology of Literary Theory and Criticism*, ed. Robyn R. Warhol and Diane Price Herndl, 417–431. New Brunswick, N.J: Rutgers University Press.

Copjec, Joan. 2002. *UMBR(a): A Journal of the Unconscious*. UMBR(a).
Copjec, Joan. 2004. *Imagine There's No Woman: Ethics and Sublimation*. The MIT Press.
Copjec, Joan. 2015. *Read My Desire: Lacan against the Historicists. Read My Desire: Lacan against the Historicists*, Radical Thinkers. London: Verso.
Copjec, Joan. 2018. The Sexual Compact. In *Sex and Nothing*, ed. Alejandro Cerda-Rueda, 1st ed., 107–137. Routledge.
Daly, Ruth. 2021. Disrupting Phallic Logic: (Re)Thinking the Feminine with Hélène Cixous and Bracha Ettinger. *Australian Feminist Studies* 36 (109): 335–351.
Ettinger, Bracha Lichtenberg. 1992. Matrix and Metramorphosis. *Differences: A Journal of Feminist Cultural Studies* 4 (3): 176–209.
Ettinger, Bracha. 1994. The Becoming Threshold of Matrixial Borderlines. In *Travellers' Tales: Narratives of Home and Displacement*, ed. George Robertson, Melinda Mash, Lisa Tickner, Jon Bird, Barry Curtis, and Tim Putnam, 36–60. London: Routledge.
Ettinger, Bracha. 1996. Metramorphic Borderlinks and Matrixial Borderspace. In *Rethinking Borders*, ed. John C. Welchman. Minneapolis: University of Minnesota Press.
Ettinger, Bracha. 1997. The Feminine/Prenatal Weaving in Matrixial Subjectivity-as-Encounter. *Psychoanalytic Dialogues* 7 (3): 367–405.
Ettinger, Bracha. 1999. "Trauma and Beauty: Trans-subjectivity in Art." In Fatal Women: Essays on Film Noir and Related Matters, edited by Kjell R Soleim, 115–28. Bergen, Norway: University of Bergen, Centre for Women's and Gender Research.
Ettinger, Bracha. 2000. Transgressing With-In-To the Feminine. In *Differential Aesthetics: Art Practices, Philosophy and Feminist Understandings*, ed. Penny Florence and Nicola Foster, 1st ed., 185–210. Routledge. https://doi.org/10.4324/9781315182735-13.
Ettinger, Bracha. 2001. Matrixial Gaze and Screen: Other Than Phallic and Beyond the Late Lacan. In *Bodies of Resistance: New Phenomenologies of Politics, Agency, and Culture*, ed. Laura Doyle, 103–143. Evanston: Northwestern University Press.
Ettinger, Bracha. 2004. Weaving a Woman Artist With-in the Matrixial Encounter-Event. *Theory, Culture & Society* 21 (1): 69–94.
Ettinger, Bracha. 2005. 'Copoiesis'. Ephemera: Theory & Politics in Organization 5(X): 703–13.
Ettinger, Bracha L. 2006a. Fascinance and the Girl-to-M/Other Matrixial Feminine Difference. In *Psychoanalysis and the Image*, ed. Griselda Pollock, 60–93. Oxford, UK: Blackwell Publishing Ltd.

Ettinger, Bracha. 2006d. *The Matrixial Borderspace. The Matrixial Borderspace*, Theory out of Bounds. Vol. 28. Minneapolis: University of Minnesota Press.

Ettinger, Bracha. 2007. Diotima and the Matrixial Transference: Psychoanalytical Encounter-Event as Pregnancy in Beauty. In *Beyond the Threshold: Explorations of Liminality in Literature*, ed. Hein Viljoen and Chris N. Van der Merwe, 105–134. New York: Peter Lang.

Ettinger, Bracha Lichtenberg. 2009a. '"Fragilization and Resistance"'. Studies in the Maternal 1 (2): 1–31. https://doi.org/10.16995/sim.141.

Ettinger, Bracha Lichtenberg. 2009b. '"Fragilization and Resistance" and "Neighborhood and Shechina"'. Studies in the Maternal 1 (2): 1–31. https://doi.org/10.16995/sim.141.

Ettinger, Bracha L. 2014b. Demeter-Persephone complex, entangled aerials of the psyche, and Sylvia Plath. ESC: English studies in Canada 40.1: 123–154.

Ettinger, Bracha Lichtenberg. 2016. 'Laius Complex and Shocks of Maternality: With Franz Kafka and Sylvia Plath'. In Interdisciplinary Handbook of Trauma and Culture, edited by Haviva Pedaya, David Gurevitz, Yuval Neria, and Yochai Ataria. Springer International Publishing.

Ettinger, Bracha Lichtenberg. 2017 Transgressing with-in-to the feminine. Differential aesthetics. Routledge, 185–210.

Ettinger, B. 2019. 'Beyond the Death-Drive, beyond the Life-Drive: Being-toward-Birthing with Being-toward-Birth; Copoiesis and the Matrixial Eros—Metafeminist Notes'. Aberrant Nuptials: Deleuze and Artistic Research, 183–214.

Fisher, R. Michael. 2024. Teaching Ettingerian Matrixial Theory. *Artizein: Arts and Teaching Journal* 9 (1): 12.

Giffney, Noreen, Anne Mulhall, and Michael O'Rourke. 2009. Seduction into Reading: Bracha L. Ettinger's The Matrixial Borderspace. *Studies in the Maternal* 1 (2): 1–15.

Greenberger, Alex. 2023. Israeli Artist Bracha L. Ettinger Resigns from Documenta 16 Selection Committee. *ARTnews*. https://www.artnews.com/art-news/news/bracha-l-ettinger-resigns-documenta-16-selection-committee-israel-1234686454/.

Gutiérrez-Albilla, Julián Daniel. 2022. Introduction: The Primary Event of Peace: Femininity, Com-Passionate Hospitality, and Aesthetic Wit(h)Nessing in Bracha L. Ettinger's Matrixial Psychoanalysis. *Psychoanalysis, Culture & Society* 27 (4): 466–484.

Johnson, Anna Louise. 2006.'Bracha Ettinger's Theory of the Matrix: Contexts and Commentary. ProQuest Dissertations & Theses.

Kinsella, Tina. 2019. A Cord That Is Never Done Away with: An Aesthetic Ontology of the Pre-Birth Scene with Francesca Woodman and Bracha L. Ettinger. In *Maternal Structures in Art: Intergenerational Discussions on Motherhood and Creative Work*, ed. Valerie Walkerdine and Elena Marchevska, 1st ed., 36–48. Routledge.

Kisiel, Anna. 2017. Dis-obedience to the Father Bracha L. Ettinger's Theory and Installation Confronted with Freud and Lacan. *Romanica Silesiana* 12:53–63.

Kisiel, Anna. 2019. Aesth/Ethical Bodies: Bracha Ettinger's Eurydices and the Encounter With the Other's History. In *The Body in History, Culture, and the Arts*, ed. Aleksandra Musiał and Justyna Jajszczok, 1st ed., 149–160. Routledge.

Kisiel, Anna. 2020. 'Gazing at Eurydice: Authorship and Otherness in Bracha L. *Ettinger'. Analyses/Rerearings/Theories (A/R/T) Journal* 6 (1): 7–17.

Kisiel, Anna. 2022. Openness in Distance: Introductory Remarks on Academic Teaching Informed by Bracha L. Ettinger's Matrixial Theory. *Studies in Philosophy and Education* 41 (5): 497–509.

Kristeva, J. 1973. The Semiotic Activity. *Screen (London)* 14 (1–2): 25–39.

Kristeva, Julia. 1980. *Desire in Language: A Semiotic Approach to Literature and Art. Desire in Language: A Semiotic Approach to Literature and Art*, European Perspectives. New York: Columbia University Press.

Lentchner, Anna. 2023. European Cultural Festivals Contend with Israeli-Palestine Polarization. ARTASIAPACIFIC. https://www.artasiapacific.com/news/european-cultural-festivals-contend-with-israel-palestine-polarization/.

MacNamara, Nóirín. 2021. Precarity and Judith Butler's Ambivalent Social Bond. What Is the Value of Ettingerian Transconnectedness? In *Precarity and International Relations*, 203–228. Springer International Publishing.

MacNamara, Nóirín. 2024. The Value of Owning the Symbols That Orientate Us within Subjectivity. *Feminist Theory* 26 (2): 426–445.

Malone, Kareen Ror. 1997. Working through the Question of the Phallus to the Other Side Commentary on Bracha Lichtenberg-Ettinger's Paper. *Psychoanalytic Dialogues* 7 (3): 407–422.

Mitchell, Juliet, and Jacqueline Rose. 1983. *Feminine Sexuality: Jacques Lacan and the École Freudienne*. London: Macmillan.

Neill, Calum. 2008. Severality: Beyond the Compression of the Cogito. *Subjectivity* 24:325–339.

Pollock, Griselda. 1992. 'Trouble in the Archives: Introduction'. *Differences: A Journal of Feminist Cultural Studies* 4 (3): iii–xiv.

Pollock, Griselda. 1994. The Work of Bracha Lichtenberg-Ettinger: An Introduction. *Third Text* 8 (28–29): 61–70.

Pollock, Griselda. 1996. The Presence of the Future: Feminine and Jewish Difference: Intricate but I Hope Not Incoherent Thoughts on Identity and Art. *Issues in Architecture, Art & Design* 5 (1).

Pollock, Griselda. 1999. Painting as a Backward Glance That Does Not Kill: Eurydice (1992–99) by Bracha Lichtenberg Ettinger. *Renaissance and Modern Studies* 42 (1): 116–144.

Pollock, Griselda. 2001. "Abandoned at the Mouth of Hell or a Second Look That Does Not Kill: The Uncanny Coming to Matrixial Memory." In Looking Back to the Future: Essays on Art, Life and Death, 113–74. Amsterdam:G+B Arts International.

Pollock, Griselda. 2004. Thinking the Feminine: Aesthetic Practice as Introduction to Bracha Ettinger and the Concepts of Matrix and Metramorphosis. *Theory, Culture & Society* 21 (1): 5–65.

Pollock, Griselda. 2005. Gleaning in History or Coming after/behind the Reapers: The Feminine, the Stranger and the Matrix in the Work and Theory of Bracha Lichtenberg Ettinger. In *Generations and Geographies in the Visual Arts: Feminist Readings*, 342–373. Routledge.

Pollok, Griselda. 2006. 'Beyond Oedipus: Feminist Thought, Psychoanalysis and Mythical Figurations of the Feminine'. In *Laughing with Medusa: Classical Myth and Feminist Thought*, edited by Vando Zajko and Miriam Leonard. Classical Presences. Oxford University Press. https://doi.org/10.1093/acprof:oso/9780199237944.001.0001.

Pollock, Griselda. 2006. Femininity: Aporia or Sexual Difference? In *The Matrixial Borderspace*, Theory out of Bounds, ed. Bracha Ettinger, vol. 28. Minneapolis: University of Minnesota Press.

Pollock, Griselda. 2007. What Does a Woman Want? Art Investigating Death in Charlotte Salomon's Leben? Oder Theater? *Art History* 30 (3): 383–405.

Pollock, Griselda. 2009a. Art/Trauma/Representation. *Parallax (Leeds, England)* 15 (1): 40–54.

Pollock, Griselda. 2009b. Mother Trouble: The Maternal-Feminine in Phallic and Feminist Theory in Relation to Bratta Ettinger's Elaboration of Matrixial Ethics. *Studies in the Maternal* 1 (1): 1–31.

Pollock, Griselda. 2013. Art as Transport-Station of Trauma? Haunting Objects in the Works of Bracha Ettinger, Sarah Kofman and Chantal Akerman. In *Representing Auschwitz: At the Margins of Testimony*, 194–221. Springer.

Pollock, Griselda. 2013. *Visual Politics of Psychoanalysis: Art and the Image in Post-Traumatic Cultures*. I.B. Tauris, London and New York.

Pollock, Griselda. 2014a. Abandoned at the Mouth of Hell or a Second Look That Does Not Kill: The Uncanny Coming to Matrixial Memory. In *Looking Back to the Future*, ed. Saul Ostrow, 1st ed., 113–174. Routledge.

Pollock, Griselda. 2014b. Sarah Kofman's Father's Pen and Bracha Ettinger's Mother's Spoon: Trauma, Transmission and the Strings of Virtuality. In *Objects and Materials*, ed. Gillian Evans, Penny Harvey, Elizabeth B. Silva, Kath Woodward, Eleanor Conlin Casella, Christine McLean, Nicholas Thoburn, and Hannah Knox, 1st ed., 162–172. Routledge.

Pollock, Griselda. 2016. Is Feminism a Trauma, a Bad Memory, or a Virtual Future? *Differences* 27 (2): 27–61.

Pollock, Griselda. 2017. The Missing Wit(h)Ness: Monroe, Fascinance and the Unguarded Intimacy of Being Dead. *Journal of Visual Art Practice* 16 (3): 265–296.

Pollock, Griselda. 2019. "Akerman" on-Screen: Chantal Akerman behind and before the Camera, and after Cinema. *Moving Image Review & Art Journal* 8 (1–2): 8–26.

Pollock, Griselda. 2023a. *Encounters in the Virtual Feminist Museum: Time, Space and the Archive*. Routledge.

Pollock, Griselda. 2023b. The Graces of Catastrophe: Matrixial Time and Aesthetic Space Confront the Archive of Disaster. In *Encounters in the Virtual Feminist Museum*, 166–198. Routledge.

Ragland, Ellie. 2008. The Masquerade, the Veil, and the Phallic Mask. *Psychoanalysis, Culture & Society* 13 (1): 8–23.

Ragland-Sullivan, Ellie. 2012. *The Logic of Sexuation: From Aristotle to Lacan. The Logic of Sexuation: From Aristotle to Lacan*, SUNY Series in Psychoanalysis and Culture. Albany: State University of New York Press.

Ragland-Sullivan, Ellie. 2014. The Sexual Masquerade: A Lacanian Theory of Sexual Difference. In *Lacan and the Subject of Language*, ed. Mark Bracher and Ellie Ragland-Sullivan, 1st ed., 49–80. Routledge.

Rank, Otto. 2015. *The Trauma of Birth*. Ravenio Books.

Rodriguez, Karen. 2016. Someone Else Is Singing through Your Throat: Language, Trauma and Bracha L. Ettinger's Wit (h) Nessing. *Critical Multilingualism Studies* 4 (1): 25–43.

Rose, Jacqueline. 2005. *Sexuality in the Field of Vision. Sexuality in the Field of Vision*, Radical Thinkers. Vol. 9. London: Verso.

Rowley, Alison. 1999. An Introduction to Bracha Lichtenberg-Ettinger's Traumatic Wit(h)Ness-Thing and Matrixial Co/in-Habit(u)Ating. *Parallax (Leeds, England)* 5 (1): 83–88.

Sander, Nina. 2024. Heartbreak and Wild Possibilities: Sublime Encounters with the Eco-Maternal. *Psychoanalytic Perspectives* 21 (3): 373–393.

Silverman, Kaja. 1992. The Lacanian Phallus. *Differences* 4 (1): 84–115.
Simon, Tracy. 2024. Mothers: Inhabiting the Impossible. *Studies in Gender and Sexuality* 25 (3): 191–198.
Smart, Genevieve. 2021. Impossible Births: Childbirth Beyond the (M)Other in Jacques Lacan and Mina Loy. *PSYART (Gainesville, Fla.)*, 1–1.
Smith, Mariëlle. 2013. Subjectivity as Encounter: Feminine Ethics in the Work of Bracha Lichtenberg-Ettinger and Anne Enright. *Hypatia* 28 (3): 633–645.
Soler, Colette. 2002a. Hysteria in Scientific Discourse. In *Reading Seminar XX: Lacan's Major Work on Love, Knowledge, and Feminine Sexuality*, SUNY Series in Psychoanalysis and Culture, ed. Suzanne Barnard and Bruce Fink. Albany, NY: State University of New York Press.
Soler, Colette. 2002b. What Does the Unconscious Know about Women. In *Reading Seminar XX: Lacan's Major Work on Love, Knowledge, and Feminine Sexuality*, SUNY Series in Psychoanalysis and Culture, ed. Suzanne Barnard and Bruce Fink. Albany, NY: State University of New York Press.
Soler, Colette. 2006. *What Lacan Said about Women: A Psychoanalytic Study*. Other Press, LLC.
Soler, Colette. 2012. Identité et sexuation. In *Désirs et sexualités*, 21–29. Érès.
Soler, Colette. 2023. *Towards Identity in the Psychoanalytic Encounter: A Lacanian Perspective*. 1st ed. Oxford: Routledge.
Solstreif-Pirker, Christoph. 2022. The Scream Is Not Silenced: A Mountainous Passage to Ettingerian Environmental Ethics. *Psychoanalysis, Culture & Society* 27 (4): 563–578.
Solstreif-Pirker, Christoph. 2023. Toward a Feminine-Matrixial Understanding of Modernity: Subjectivity-as-World-Fabric, the Ecology of Love, and the Temporality of Just Now. *Comparative Literature Studies (Urbana)* 60 (3): 561–577.
Torre, Shanna de la. 2018. *Sex for Structuralists: The Non-Oedipal Logics of Femininity and Psychosis*. Cham, Switzerland: Palgrave Macmillan.
Van Loo, Sofie. 2009. Colourline Painting by Bracha L. Ettinger: The Transject as Abstract-Realist Artwork in an Analogue-Dialogue with the (Un) Heimliche. *Studies in the Maternal* 1 (2).
Vigneault, Marissa. 2011. The Porous Space of Bracha Ettinger's Eurydices. In *Contemporary Art and Classical Myth*, 111–133. Ashgate: Publishing.
Voela, Angie. 2014. Wit (h) Finessing the Other's Trauma. In *The Ethics of Remembering and the Consequences of Forgetting: Essays on Trauma, History, and Memory*, New Imago: Series in Theoretical, Clinical, and Applied Psychoanalysis, ed. Michael O'Loughlin. Lanham: Rowman & Littlefield.

Voela, Angie, and Cigdem Esin. 2021. Movement, Embrace: Adriana Cavarero with Bracha Lichtenberg Ettinger (and the Death Drive). *Hypatia* 36 (1): 101–119.

Walsh, Fintan. 2011. From Enthusiasm to Encounter-Event: Bracha L. Ettinger, Samuel Beckett and the Theatre of Affect. *Parallax (Leeds, England)* 17 (2): 110–123.

Wierzchowska, Justyna. 2022. Creating Together an "Unexpected Home": Navigating the Matrixial Borderspace Through Text and Image in Mary Kelly's Post-Partum Document (1973–79). In *Text and Image in Women's Life Writing*, Palgrave Studies in Life Writing, 259–277. Cham: Springer International Publishing.

Zajko, Vanda, and Miriam Leonard, eds. 2006. Laughing with Medusa: Classical Myth and Feminist Thought. OUP Oxford.

Zupančič, Alenka. 2017. *What IS Sex?* Short Circuits. 1st ed. Cambridge: The MIT Press.

2

The Matrixial Borderspace

Bracha L. Ettinger contends that psychoanalytic theories of human subjectivity are limited to the extent that they focus on the early years of life after-birth while neglecting pre-birth experience. Without attention to pregnancy and gestation, the central importance of what Ettinger calls the matrixial borderspace is eclipsed. In this chapter, I outline her critique of Freud and Lacan who, in Ettinger's assessment, negate intrauterine experience. I then provide an overview of Ettinger's theory of the matrixial borderspace with attention to four critical components of her theorization: matrixial subjectivity; *metra*morphosis; the matrixial gaze; and the borderlinking. Following this, I situate Ettinger's theory of the matrixial in relation to the feminist writings of Luce Irigaray and Julia Kristeva who also respond to Lacan's writing on the mother and the Feminine. I do so to illustrate Ettinger's unique contribution to theorizing Feminine difference and the mother from the perspective of the matrixial borderspace. Let us begin with Ettinger's critique of Freud and Lacan so that we can more fully appreciate and contextualize her scholarly contribution to psychoanalysis.

Ettinger contends that Freud and Lacan were reticent to theorize intrauterine experience along with its relevance to the psychic life of the

S. L. Cavanagh, *Bracha L. Ettinger and Jacques Lacan*, The Palgrave Lacan Series,
https://doi.org/10.1007/978-3-032-23293-9_2

subject. For example, in his writing on the uncanny, Freud speculates that the fear of being buried alive is a transformation of an earlier, more primal phantasy of being in utero. Ettinger explains that body memories of being with-in-Feminine-difference are, for Freud, terrifying when recalled at a later post-Oedipal developmental stage. These memories challenge the Oedipal-boy's healthy narcissism and bind him (regressively) to the mother. Ettinger challenges the Freudian formulation of the uncanny and the boy's need to forget (repress) phantasies involving pre-uterine experience. She counters that an object is not uncanny by definition, but that it can be regressive and scary when it cannot be represented. The maternal object is not, by definition, harmful but the trace of the m/Other can be threatening to a phallic subject when the Feminine dimension of difference is foreclosed as an avenue of expression. It is, for Ettinger, imperative to find ways of expressing and giving form to the Feminine dimension of difference so that matrixial links to Others can be apprehended.

The ego is, for Freud, first and foremost a bodily ego. To the extent that our relations to the bodily organs of the m/Other are foreclosed in phantasy, there is a lack of integration of the Feminine-matrixial. Ettinger puts it thus: "Relations to bodily organs that are not integrated into the perception of the whole object…are all experiences of no return leading to a veiled acknowledgement of a certain failure inherent in the [phallic] relations toward Otherness" (2006c, 62).

The failure on the part of the phallic relation to otherness is, for Ettinger, due to a negation of the matrixial-Feminine. In the matrixial we all apprehend un-cognized memories and phantasies involving the mother that must be apprehended and expressed as Ettinger does through her art-practice (2000, 2011, 2015). The Eros of the matrixial-borderlinking is not a threat to the subject but what enables a dimension of subjectivity involving others and otherness. Transitivism is thus central to the Feminine, but not regressive; it is core to a non-Oedipal sexual difference in the braiding of the Real and the Imaginary. The signifier does not reign in this orbit of sexual difference. As such, it cannot be directly signified. For Ettinger, it follows that the Lacanian Symbolic fails to grasp bodily and psychical phenomena relating to the matrixial borderspace.

It must also be stressed that this orbit of Feminine difference predates gender identity, sexual orientation (in the phallic dimension), kinship systems, and language. Ettinger contends that the Feminine-matrixial bears no relation to sexual positioning in Lacanian terms, but we may, in my interpretation of it, better understand what Lacan calls the Other (Feminine) jouissance through her theorization of the matrixial (as I will discuss in later chapters).

The Matrixial Borderspace

For Ettinger, the matrixial borderspace is irreducible to legal jurisprudence and cannot be understood within its terms: it involves another ethic dramatized in Sophocles' *Antigone*. As we know from the Oedipal trilogy which figures prominently in the history of psychoanalysis, Antigone is steadfast in her opposition to Creon's Law governing kinship structures in the city of Thebes. As I explain in Chap. 7, Antigone's devotion or, in Ettinger's terms, borderlinking, to her brother predates and exceeds the law of the land. He must be buried in Theban soil despite the King forbidding it. In order to understand what is at stake in the feminist tragedy that has enchanted audiences, psychoanalysts, and legal scholars alike, we must consider elements of being, relating to the Feminine dimension of difference, that are unspeakable, yet salient. In order to understand the Feminine realm of experience including trauma, desire, Eros, and jouissance relating to it, Ettinger posits a theory of the matrixial borderspace to account for our borderlinkings to Others (as *non-I*'s).

As intimated above, the matrixial borderspace is based on unremembered and un-cognized experiences in utero where (and when) we cannot be without the mother as first Other. The becoming-subject in utero and the becoming-mother who is pregnant exist in complex relations that enable co-emergence and differentiation. The unremembered and phantasmatic borderspace of co-emergence in utero are psychically invested in adult life. Trace-like memories of a shared body-space in the womb are unconscious but they, nevertheless, give form to a Feminine dimension of difference relevant to everyone, regardless of gender or sexuation in later life. The Feminine dimension of difference theorized by Ettinger is not specific to cisgender women; it is felt and negotiated by everyone regardless of gender and sexual positioning in the phallic dimension.

While Ettinger theorizes female reproductive capacity and the sexuating encounter-event of gestation and birth, she uses the matrix as a metaphor to conceptualize Real and Imaginary components of the Feminine-matrixial dimension. The matrix is not a symbol and it does not replace the phallus. Ettinger writes that that the "matrix is no more – but no less – related to the womb than the phallus is related to the penis" (Ettinger 1993, 12). As Griselda Pollock explains, "Matrix 'thinks' pregnancy/pre-birth as structure (not a body or a place and never an organ – organ thinking is phallic)" (2013, 168). Likewise, there is no placenta and no womb to be taken as separate from the Real and Imaginary. The matrix is not a flesh-like thing or signifiable space or essence in Ettingerian vocabulary. Female corporeality matters in Ettinger's theory of the matrixial but it is not a material substrate separable from phantasy, desire, aesthetics, affects, time, memory, etc.

Matrixial theory is modeled upon experiences of pregnancy and gestation, the fetus, and the womb as a "conceptual basis for a difference that takes into consideration a corpo-Real dimension" (Ettinger 2006c, 179). The corpo-Real can be understood as an assemblage that interweaves the Real and the sensory, aesthetic and corporeal schemata of the body. The matrixial is a Feminine place of co-emergence, severalty, and becoming. As Ettinger explains, the matrixial is a "complex apparatus modeled on this site of feminine-prenatal encounter…that places any human becoming-subject-to-be, male or female, in relation with female bodily specificity" (141). Equally, the matrixial, like pregnancy, is not based on fusion or symbiosis. It involves complex functions, aesthetics, affects, objects, and trace-like memories that bind us to our others whom she calls our *non-I*'s (or partners in difference). The Other is not a separate subject, but a partial-subject in matrixial terms. Likewise, the *non-I* is part of the subject. Both the *I* and *non-I* exist in shared psychic spaces where there is contiguity without symmetry. Let us be clear that the Ettingerian subject is not One, but several, and this is why she speaks of partial-subjectivity, as opposed to individual subjectivity as such.

The Other co-affects and lives alongside the self, as partial-subject. In the matrixial sub-stratum, the "I disappears so that the Other will arrive"

(Ettinger 2006b, 114). The matrixial borderspace enables the *I* and the *non-I* to transform and to differentiate. Part of what occurs in the border-linking is a registration of a metramorphic link involving the *I* and *non-I*. Through affective re-attunements in the matrixial web, the *I* and *non-I* share a borderspace that allows both — and multiple others known and unknown in the same web — to co-fade and to co-emerge without similitude. Even in solitude, one cannot be without their copoietic *non-I*'s. "The I is a pulsating pole of co-poiesis. The *I* and *non-I* are pulsating poles of co-poiesis along a shared psychic string" (Ettinger 2006c, 193). Copoiesis refers to a transformational potentiality in the matrixial. It is not semiotic in Kristevian terms, or based on fusion. It is, ultimately, aesthetic and ethical.[1]

Matrixial Subjectivity

Ettinger's formulation of the matrixial borderspace is based on a model of subjectivity whereby we exist in relation to others in a phantasmatic field. The matrixial borderspace is an ever-changing space-event of cross-pollination whereby two or more partial-subjects encounter and co-affect each other in non-conscious ways. In order to grasp the significance of Ettinger's proposition regarding the partial-subject as several, it is first necessary to rethink our preconceptions about transitivity.

Transitivism is usually understood either in relation to Freud's theory of a child being beaten whereby a child who witnesses a beating imagines that it is they who are beaten, or in relation to the Lacanian mirror stage where Lacan talks about "normal transitivism" that occurs between six and thirty months of age. For Lacan, there is a structural ambivalence associated with the mirror stage. As he discusses in his "Presentation on Psychical Causality", the mirror stage is associated with what he calls a "primordial ambivalence" (147), with the way the Other's desire becomes central to our ideal ego (2006c 571), and with aggression. While

[1] Ettinger distinguishes between autopoiesis and copoiesis. The former relates to the cellular structure whereby the *non-I* is an object. Copoiesis is an "affective humanizing alliance of differences, difference-in-jointness, and differentiation in co-emergence that calls for sensuality and sensibility, affective arousal and emotional cathexis, and human care: communicaring".

transitivism is usually understood as specific to a developmental stage and thought to be regressive when experienced in adulthood, it is, for Ettinger, a basis for matrixial ethics. Far from being regressive or infantile, transitivism is, from the perspective of the matrixial, what enables empathy, compassion, fragility, and shared traumata (Ettinger 2006b, 2007, 2011).

In Ettingerian terms, transitivity is about subjectivity as encounter (or severality). When Ettinger refers to partial-subjectivity, she is referring to a formation of subjectivity whereby the Other is not separate or alien, but borderlinked to the I. For Lacanians it may be helpful to recall that he also refers to the I as an Other in his notes on the unconscious. But Ettinger maps out this subjective equation in more elaborate detail through her theory of the matrixial. For her, transitivity involves transmissivity and co-affectivity. It is not about *having* or *being* the phallus, for example, but about the unthought time-space of borderlinking in the Real. Moreover, the transitive sexual difference of relevance to Ettinger is not about fusion, symbiosis, regression, or rejection. Transitivity is about the sharing and transmission of differentiated objects through archaic traces and borderlinks (Ettinger 2006c).

For Ettinger, the subject is not One (or whole) in the matrixial axis of difference, but more than one (transitive). We exist in relation to others (*non-I's*) in the matrixial borderspace. As such, we co-emergence, separate, and differentiate in non-conscious and asymmetrical relations. In order to explicate her theory of matrixial transitivity, Ettinger develops specific terminology relating to partial-subjectivity (synonymous with severality). There are two main components to partial-subjectivity: the sub-subjective and the trans-subjective. The sub-subjective involves an aggregated subjectivity and the trans-subjective involves our relations to uncognized *non-I's* and others. The trans-subjective is a matrixial variant on the transitional object posited by Winnicott and *object a* by Lacan. "The ideas of transitional object and space, like those of the 'third,' contribute to what I have come to recognize as trans(sub)jectivity. Its symbolic understanding – in-betweenness that is not a third or transitional space and object and metramorphosis – demands metaphoric approximations" (Ettinger 2016, 288). By the trans-subjective plain, Ettinger is referring to relations between partial-subjects and partial-objects composed of links, traces and webs, as opposed to castrating cuts, phallic knots, and relations between individuated subjects. On occasion, she also uses the term "trans-relationality" and "transconnectivity" (Ettinger 2009, 18).

In psychoanalytic theory, references are made to intersubjectivity. But, in Ettingerian theory, it makes sense to speak about intra-subjectivity because traumas, desires, experiences and phantasmatic relations are significant to life with non-cognized Others. Intra-subjectivity is not, for Ettinger, based on fusion or symbiosis. Her theory represents a departure from psychoanalytic approaches akin to those developed by Christopher Bollas who, for instance, understands the late intrauterine encounter in terms of symbiosis and "psychosomatic sensations of *fusion*" (Ettinger 2006c, 78). Ettinger's theory explicates how this encounter is, in fact, subjectivizing and discernable in the sub-Symbolic. In the matrixial field, "*subsymbolic processes of interconnectivity*" (64) are not only possible but signifiable.

Our attunement to Others and *non-Is* is, for Ettinger, intra-subjective because they are based on linkages in a shared phantasmatic body-space. The shared body-space in a given matrixial web resonates and affects us all as co-emerging partial-subjects in a weave or matrixial net. We are not (only) One (in the phallic sense) but several in the matrixial (Feminine) axis of difference. Ettinger writes about subjectivity *as encounter* in a way that harkens back to phantasies in uterine that reverberate in the corpo-Real and linked to phantasy. Ettinger will sometimes refer to a "dispersal and loss of the self" (Ettinger 2009) in the sub-subjective psychic space which cannot be understood in intersubjective terms alone. This is to say that there is a "Self-with-other psychic dimension of subjectivity" (Ettinger 2006c, 82) that is irreducible to individual subjects, and to intersubjectivity more generally.

Recall that the matrixial borderspace is a phantasmatic field where (and when) the I exists in relation to Others and *non-Is* as partners-in-difference. Ettinger names this phantasmatic field the sub-Symbolic as distinct from the Lacanian Symbolic. As noted above, the matrixial sub-Symbolic involves the Real, the Imaginary, and what Ettinger calls a broadened Symbolic. The matrixial sub-Symbolic resonates in and alters the Lacanian Symbolic. Ettinger writes: "*Sub*symbolic matrixial processes are interwoven into the Symbolic and change it from within" (2006c,

64). These matrixial processes are subjacent, not anterior and need not remain unsymbolizable or pre-symbolic. The sub-symbolic dimension is outside the tentacles of the phallic organ (as signifier) and the image (as imaginary referent). But they, nevertheless, exist in the matrixial-Feminine dimension.

Ettinger is critical of the way the woman and the mother are reduced to *object a* (object cause of desire) and to *das Ding* (the *Thing*) in Lacanian theory. She thus develops a feminist supplement through her formulation of the *a-link*. The matrixial *a-link* gives theoretical form to the phantasmatic field where the m/Other and the woman are not reducible to objects, radical Others, or things. *a-links* are comparable to psychic strings binding a given matrixial web. They enable matrixial subjects to apprehend Real and phantasmatic apparitions. In other words, there is something sensorial or telepathic that resonates with the aggregated subject. An *a-link* is also what Ettinger calls the "trace of a borderlinking" (2006c, 56). It is closely related to what she calls an erotic aerial which apprehends the Other's traces. An erotic aerial is best understood as a string or psychic wire through which partial-subjects apprehend matrixial affects in distance and proximity to others.

Within a given resonance field, certain *a-links* become more pronounced and, consequently, structure the web in such a way that it is marked by the vibrations, frequencies, repetitions and intensities of those particular psychic strings. Each string stores a memory shared by *I* and *non-I*'s and Others who co-emerge and borderlink in a given web. Traces of each thread are felt within each partial subject through a-links. Each web has its own unique composition of trace-like threads that get re-knitted in the time-space of the metramorphic encounter-event. The *a-link* enables matrixial affects. Matrixial affects are "shaped and transformed by feminine trauma and phantasy linked to female bodily specificity on the level of the Real" (2006c, 84). Ettinger explains how matrixial affects are like psychical engravings. She also describes them as inscriptions that borderlink the I to unknown others and as core to the "trans-subjective matrixial alliance" (Ettinger 2001, 128).

As Ettinger explains, matrixial affective links enable us to transgress to the "m/Other via the eroticized antennae of the psyche" (2006c, 56). She (1996) further notes that "passages are made between the matrixial stratum and the phallic stratum in the same subject" (153). These passages can be understood if "alongside traces of objects – we conceive of traces of links and relations, from the angle of a *co-emerging I and non-I* prior to the *I versus others*" (Ettinger 2006c, 64).

This is, in part, what enables her to argue contra Lacan that there is a sexual relation from the perspective of the matrixial, if not from the perspective of the phallic premise. Let us remember that Lacan challenges the idea that there is a sexual relationship between men and women. By this, he means that the phallic (masculine) jouissance and the Other (feminine) jouissance are asymmetrical and have nothing to do with each other. But as we will see in chapters to follow, there is a sexual relation from the perspective of the matrixial.

It should also be noted that the time of the matrixial is non-linear. It is elliptic and future-oriented. Although Ettinger says the matrixial subject knows that there is a future (and past) without me, the matrixial borderlinking is not best understood as harmonious or utopic: it can be terrifying and traumatizing because one risks fragmentation and regression. The matrixial is not a cozy covenant but a multilayered webbing of Others and *non-I*'s with and for whom the subject exists. Referring to matrixial co-subjectivity, Pollock writes that it is the "pathway of transmitted trauma, hatred, anxiety, or fear" (Pollock 2008, 32) as much as it can be a grounding for ethics. Matrixial encounter-events must also be understood in these terms. Ettinger explains that the matrixial Thing is like an archaic jouissance (although it is ultimately healing, life affirming and futuristic). As Ettinger explains, the "desire to join-in-difference and differentiate-in-co-emergence with the Other…[involves] a joining within the other's trauma that echoes back to my archaic traumas" (2006c, 147). Sharing by joining in difference and differentiating in co-emergence is profoundly unsettling insofar as it threatens us with mental disintegration and memory of oblivion. As Ettinger explains, "The potential is there for traumatic and destructive as well as ethical or aesthetic deposits of jouissance" (2006c, 18). We are all subject to trauma and jouissance in the matrixial and the resultant trace inscriptions and crypts.

Ettinger is apt to illustrate the traumatic legacies resulting from injustice to, or disrespect for, matrixial links in Greek tragedies and in Hebrew scripture. She explains that when "manipulative appropriation or controlling humiliation arise, the borderlines that function as borderlinking thresholds can also inform autistic boundaries and transform into autistic boundaries" (Ettinger 2009, 13). Ettinger also comments upon the problem of meeting primary compassion with "abandonment" or "engulfment" in the matrixial borderspace (17). "Thantos wins when the web of borderlinks is shattered into endless fragments, and when it evaporates or liquidates itself into fusion or when a subject/object split [that is phallic] takes over" (17). In later chapters, I use Ettinger's work on borderlinking in the familial web to illustrate what counts not only as Oedipal tragedy, but matrixial trauma in the Freudian case study of Dora, the character of Lol Stein in the Marguerite Duras novel, and in *Antigone*.

The familial webs central to the three female characters are Real (in Lacanian terms), but they can be apprehended. As Ettinger contends, matrixial traumas leave non-signifying imprints in the Symbolic. The "matrixial web of severality includes remnants of jouissance and trauma: imprints of whoever was there, as subknowledge that is not just traces of lack but also trails of what is beyond and yet inter-with-in me" (Ettinger 2001, 131). This Feminine sub-knowledge is not about what is lacking, but rather about what is "beyond and yet inter-with-in me" (131). The "beyond" (trans-subjective) and "inter-with-in me" (sub-subjective) is, as already noted, predicated upon Ettinger's specific reinterpretation of Lacan's original notes on transitivism. Feminine sex difference is, for Ettinger, about transitivism, but transitivism with a metramorphic difference.

Metramorphosis

In order to theorize change in the borderlinking, Ettinger reformulates the Lacanian reference to metamorphosis in matrixial terms. *Metra*morphosis is a process involving change, what Deleuze and Guattari (1987) would call "becomings." But unlike the Deleuzian and Guattarian notion of becoming, Ettinger's use of the term is bound by the texture and specificity of a given matrixial web. For Ettinger, becoming is generative, erotic, and future-oriented. It involves rhizomatic movements and transmogrifications but these shape-shifting experiences are unique and particular to each partial-subject and thus to each matrixial weave. Likewise, the matrix is "neither Nothing, nor One, nor Infinite" (Ettinger 1996, 127). Ettinger positions Deleuze and Guattari's writing on rhizomatic connectedness in the phallic stratum because their notion of the feminine is anti-Oedipal. The "anti" places their feminine difference in the phallic stratum *as* a contrast, whereas Feminine difference in the matrixial stratum refers to another dimension entirely.

Ettinger refers to metramorphosis as a "noncastrative process of passability and conductivity, repression and dispersal that creates transformations-in-differentiation and makes sense beyond distinct representations and discourse" (Ettinger 1997, 368). Ettinger also defines metramorphosis as a process of "joining-in-separating with/from the other" (Ettinger 2001, 104). In the joining-in-separating, there is a mental, affective, and emotional swerving in, to, and with the other. The process of separation in jointness, borderlinking while differentiating (2006b, 114) is subjectifying and not, as Ettinger explains, based on fusion or symbiosis.

Metramorphosis is not only transformative, but transgressive. It has transformative potential but is also about co-fading. It is an intrapsychic and interpsychic phenomenon that is transindividual. Ettinger describes metramorphosis as a poietic involving "affective-emotional swerving" (Ettinger 2006c, 182). Through a metramorphic event-encounter, there is a "joint awakening of unthoughtful-knowledge on the borderline, as well as an inscription of the encounter in traces that open a space in and along the borderline itself" (182).

In Ettinger's theory of the matrixial, metramorphosis involves copoietic changes in borderlines and thresholds, "borderlinking and distance-in-joining" (Ettinger 2000, 188). Matrixial links are central to the metramorphic process which, for Ettinger, involves a "nonpsychotic yet *beyond-the-phallus* connection between the feminine and creation" (Ettinger 2006c, 64). Metramorphosis is, in other words, a term Ettinger uses to name changes in being that involve Others and *non-I*'s in the register of the Real. While these changes also affect the Symbolic and the Imaginary, they are at the heart of a sexual difference in the Feminine dimension. As I will discuss in the following chapter, there is, for Ettinger, a "sexual difference in the Real" (51). But suffice here to say that metramorphosis may be understood as a matrixial supplement to the Lacanian reliance on metaphor and metamorphosis, which are based on substitution and contiguity respectively.

Metaphor and metonymy in Lacan's theorization work through language and discourse in the Symbolic. Metramorphosis, by contrast, refers to the generation of knowledge outside language and discourse, beyond (and before) the Symbolic. The changes in borderlines and thresholds are established through un-cognized linkages with Others and *non-I*'s. In her chapter titled "The With-In-Visible Screen," Ettinger defines metramorphosis in terms of "specific routes of passability, transmissibility, transitivity, temporary conductivity, and transference between various psychic strata, between the subject and several other subjects, and between subjects and composite hybrid objects—routes through which 'woman,' which is not the preserve of women alone, is inscribed in a subsymbolic web, knitted just-in-to the edges of a symbolic universe that cannot appropriate her in its preestablished signifiers" (94).

As I will discuss more fully in Chap. 4, Ettinger's notion of Woman is not synonymous with gender identity, natal sex, or even with the Lacanian Woman who does not exist. The Ettingerian Woman is a complex border-creature involving more than one *non-I* co-emerging in a shared border-space. Ettinger also refers to Woman as a "*border-Other*, a *becoming in-ter-with the Other*, an *im-pure becoming-between in jointness*" (2001, 72). In the Feminine zone "Woman" emerges—not as a unitary figure, but as an intricate weave trans-connecting two (or more) partial-subjects. "The matrixial stratum draws a phenomenological field of I with/for *some* other(s)" (Ettinger 2006c, 116). It may also be helpful to remember that Woman is a condition of transitivity, "not just object or subject but the structure of transitivity" (Ettinger 2004, 46). This transitivity is not about subject and object confusion, but metramorphosis involving differentiation and affective re-tuning and re-connections with Others in a given matrixial web. Matrixial desire for borderlinking is, ultimately, about copoietic change.

There is, thus, a Feminine Eros particular to the metramorphic borderlinking. Ettinger describes matrixial Eros as another kind of life-drive. It "relates to the transgenerational as well as the horizontal transmissibility of traces of memory and oblivion to what was affected in/by the individual between birth and death" (Ettinger, Beyond the Death-Drive, Beyond the Life-Drive, 10). In her article on life beyond the death drive, Ettinger notes that matrixial Eros is a "humanizing factor of difference working in relation to objects and subject-matters, caring for humans and non-human animals, for earth and for nature" (13). As such, matrixial Eros is distinct from the Lacanian theorization of desire which involves *object a* and the formative role of the Other's desire.

Matrixial desire for borderlinking is not to be confused with maternal engulfment or the crocodile mother of Lacan. It is not about amalgamation or similitude but co-emergence in differentiation. Ettinger refers to a non-genital Feminine Eros of "relations and connections which is an attraction and repulsion beyond the [Oedipal] sexual" (2007, 128). Repulsion in matrixial desire is also not about abjection in Kristeva (2024) terms, but transgression and reconfiguration. It is a borderlinking set in motion by non-phallic matrixial incest to be discussed in the following chapter. Matrixial desire is to borderlink and to differentiate within a "transgressive encounter-event and for the entirety of movements which create and fulfill such encounter-events, which, in passing by transformation would leave imprints for upcoming later transgressive encounter-events" (Ettinger 2007, 119).

One of Ettinger's most important arguments is that these transgressive encounter-events are sexual. This sexuality is not to be confused with incest in phallic terms or sexual abuse. Eros in the matrixial encounter is subjectifying, as distinct from after-birth incest which is traumatizing. While there is, in the Lacanian paradigm, only one axis of sexual difference bound by the phallic premise, there is, in Ettingerian theory, an Other Sexual Difference (OSD) that predates sexuation. Ettinger explains that there is an erotic "link to the experience of woman…[While there is] no contact with [the] feminine-Other in the sexual relationship based on the phallic model of male *jouissance* in both sexes, and most important there is no way to report on a sexual relation that would be feminine-Other if/where it does occur, since it is not inscribed in the Symbolic and no formula can sustain it" (Ettinger 2006c, 102).

The Matrixial Gaze

In order to theorize Eros in the borderlinking, Ettinger posits a matrixial gaze. The matrixial gaze is founded upon a careful reading of the Lacanian gaze where Ettinger notices that the Lacanian gaze is not altogether alienating. The screen that separates the subject from the alienating gaze of the Other is also a node of contact with the Other. The screen is not shaped by the optical laws of science, but a product of the libido. As both Ettinger and Lacan agree, there is nothing empirical about it. The screen is a libidinally cathected and phantasmatic phenomenon. It has little to do with vision per se. The visual screen is more akin to phantasy. As Lacan explains, the screen separates the gaze and the desiring subject. But for Ettinger, the gaze is also a point of contact that must be elaborated from the Feminine side.

While the matrixial gaze is predicated upon theoretical coordinates developed by Lacan, Ettinger is critical of how his formulation is developed from the perspective of the One (masculine-man) as spectator. As Ettinger summarizes in her critique of the Lacanian formulation of the gaze, the phallic gaze effectively "turns us into a picture to be looked at in phantasy, in which we do not appear to ourselves – except as a stain in the picture, or as a screen between the gaze and the picture, or as a stain on the screen" (2006c, 98). The m/Other disappears and we appear alone (as One). In Ettinger's view, the Lacanian gaze is governed by a logic of the One that involves castrating cuts, severance from the m/Other. It is founded upon an archaic split between the subject and the m/Other which, in turn, generates desire. As I will explain more fully in what follows, the gaze is one formation of Lacan's *object a* (non-object cause of desire). The gaze is, for Ettinger, a "leftover of an ancient split [from the archaic m/Other] and a surplus bygone *jouissance*" (115). Given the emphasis Lacan places on the gaze/cause of desire (a defining feature of masculine jouissance), Ettinger maintains that his formation is predicated upon "male sexual difference, experience, body and narcissism, and therefore establishes a one-sided psychic perspective" (Ettinger 2001, 117).

Ettinger's matrixial gaze is non-phallic. But she finds its theoretical coordinates in Lacan's original theorization of the gaze. Indeed, Ettinger credits Lacan for revealing that "relations are possible between a subject and another subject who looks at him/her without being observed" (Ettinger 2006c, 55). While Lacan may not have endorsed this interpretation, Ettinger finds the coordinates of a matrixial gaze in the phantom of the m/Other who lies outside of the cultural screen. For Ettinger, she is the "invisible heart of the visible" (Ettinger 2001, 116) in the gaze that Lacan sometimes calls the "tableau." There is, in other words, a "contact-mediation dimension of the screen" (115) that leaves a ghostly (matrixial) imprint (or *a-link*). For Ettinger, we project left-overs from an "archaic split and a surplus of an archaic jouissance" (32) onto the cultural screen. This is, for her, a matrixial effect insofar as it surreptitiously inscribes a-link on-in-to the cultural screen.

To explain this in another way, Ettinger agrees with Lacan that the gaze and the subject are created by a split and that there is a partition (screen). But for Ettinger, the screen is a "veil of contact whereby the gaze and the gazed-at meet and touch" (2001, 115). This leads her to question whether Lacan's gaze (as a pure *object a*) is entirely cut (or severed from the Other). It may be more haptic; a touching kind of matrixial *object a*.

Ettinger contends that a particular kind of gaze, a touching-matrixial gaze, can insert itself into the screen. The touching gaze is in the "*beyond-the-phallus* dimension" (2006c, 42). It is, for Ettinger, an affective synergy that moves beyond the "hole in being" theorized by Lacan. "The affected synergetic move/touch-and-gaze is a supplementary kind of (*a*) inasmuch as move/touch-and-gaze implies an archaic link" (Ettinger 2001, 136). This is linked to feeling-knowledge of co-affectation and trans-sensing (affective and unconscious ties between the *I* and others). Knowledge of the matrixial is what Ettinger excavates through her analytic of the gaze. Lacan agrees that there is "knowledge in the Real, which functions without us being able to know how the connection is made in what we are used to seeing happen" (Lacan quoted in Ettinger 2006a, 83). But Ettinger gives language to this knowledge in/of the Real. Moreover, she articulates how the matrixial gaze finds its way into the screen, a screen that becomes a web "into which subjectivity is woven" (Ettinger 2006c, 118).

Recall that for Ettinger the phallic gaze, as understood by Lacan, lacks reciprocity: "any mutuality between the gazed-at/seer-as-subject-also-visible-as-object (that is to say, me) and the *gaze* of the Other is illusory and every encounter is a miss" (Ettinger 2001, 98). What Ettinger adds to the Lacanian formulation is a unidirectional move that enables contact (a touching gaze) through dispersion and fragmentation. In Ettinger's definition, the matrixial gaze is a dispersion that requires the eye to "multifocalize" (139). It functions as "fission and segregation, exchange and intersection, transgression and transitivity" (135). Ettinger explains that the matrixial gaze, unlike the phallic gaze, "enters and alters the screen of vision which by definition is im-pure and inseparable from other unconscious dimensions of the psyche, informed by different sources of sensibilities, and mainly, connected to and affected by the unconscious of the Other and the consciousness of the Cosmos" (2005, 710). The non-object intercepted can never be apprehended in its entirety. Unlike the phallic gaze that can be objectifying, there is no center in the matrixial gaze and thus no object as such. "Fractions of the gaze will glint at one participant, other fractions will be received by another, and also in-between alongside the threads of the web" (Ettinger 2001, 138).

From the vantage point of the matrixial, the *object a* can be an *a-link* (a trace of an absent presence in the painting-mirror). *A-links* do not sever or cut ties; they are borderlinking events central to the OSD. While Lacan understands the gaze (that is an *object a*) to result from a cut by the signifier it is, for Ettinger, a corpo-Real cut. It is a significance that separates us from the Real of the m/Other. The gaze, from a matrixial angle is, as Ettinger suggests, a "leftover of inaccessible 'bodily samplings,' of my corpo-Reality and of the Other" (2006c, 124). This is to say that *a-link* is "a trace of borderlinking" (56) where an encounter with an Other is possible. This encounter is at the heart of the matrixial borderspace where the OSD resides makes what Ettinger calls feeling-sense.

To summarize, this matrixial *object a* (or *a-link*) is established before sexual positioning in Lacanian terms. There is, through *a-link*, a hole in the Real which enables an image of an Other to emerge. For Ettinger, *a-link* is a "touching gaze" (87). It is thus haptic as opposed to alienating. It is a "trail of separation-in-jointness that is not an incision or a cut from the archaic m/Other" (125). This separation-in-jointness is a co-affecting relation in the matrixial.

The innovative point made by Ettinger is that the Lacanian *object a* has a "borderline visibility" (Ettinger 1996, 150). By this, she means that the derivatives of the lost maternal object which includes female corpo-Reality as fragmented and dispersed objects, have a presence in phantasy. "In the invisible screen of phantasy, the *object a* is a non-specular object situated at the borderline of the subject's mirror images which are created by the Other" (150). In other words, what lacks a signifier appears in the phantasy screen invisible to the naked eye. These non-visible appearances in the screen of phantasy are access points to the OSD. While they are not delimited by what is given (in the mirror) to be seen, they are sensed and felt in the borderlinking with the m/Other.

The matrixial gaze helps Ettinger to theorize the unseen borderlinking relevant to the Feminine. In her view, we need to give form to a mode of seeing that is not only relevant to the Feminine, but to the mother as first Other. The Other (Feminine) sexual difference "produces for men and women a different, non-Oedipal sublimation where, in the search for *non-I*(s), the *jouissance* is of the borderlinking itself" (Ettinger 2001, 110). It is felt "in/by the Real" (Ettinger 1997, 401). The borderlinking is an encounter-event in the Real at the basis of Feminine sexual difference. The Feminine is an "irreducible difference *inside* subjectivity" (Ettinger 2004, 84). It is a non-phallic and non-Oedipal trans-sensitivity available to everyone. There are no individuals in the matrixial, only partial-subjects, borderlinkings, becomings, co-fadings, and metramorphosis, which are felt within the sphere of the matrixial. This is why the OSD is not specific to cisgender women, it is felt and experienced by everyone, regardless of gender identity and sexual positioning.

In her discussion of Ettinger's work on the OSD, Griselda Pollock speculates that Feminine desire might "signify something of profound importance for discussions of human subjectivity and indeed sociality" (Ettinger 2006c, 22). Here the Feminine is conceived of as a matrixial relation, a life-generating borderlinking based on un-cognized memories of the mother-to-be/subject-to-be encounter felt by those who will later become men and women. The Feminine is not set up in opposition to the masculine, to natal male sex specificity, or to transgender identity. As Ettinger explains, her formulation of the Feminine-matrixial is "not opposed to femininity in the phallic one, neither is it derived from it, nor from its masculinity; it is an originary and primordial difference" (1997, 370). Equally, the Ettingerian Feminine is not reducible to the Other Feminine jouissance theorized by Lacan, much less the Woman who is not-all inscribed in the (phallic) Symbolic. Ettinger's formulation of the Feminine (as distinct from femininity) builds upon Lévinas. It is the "irreducible difference inside subjectivity: precisely what makes it human" (Ettinger 2006c, 190). The Feminine is, in other words, the inter-human as opposed to the phallic One.

Lacanian readers may understand the Ettingerian Feminine in relation to the unconscious which he defines as trans-individual. But for Ettinger, the Feminine is better understood in terms of transitivity. In their discussion of Ettinger's feminist thought and mythology, Vanda Zaijko and Miriam Leonard (2006) explain that the Feminine is an "inter/trans-subjectivizing structure/encounter/space where potentially human subjects co-emerge and co-transform" (30). It is, in other words, a dimension and condition of plurality and difference relevant to the subject-as-several (or severality).

As such, Ettinger's theorization is central to feminist psychoanalysis and needs to be contextualized in relation to Luce Irigaray and Julia Kristeva who have also reformulated Lacanian ideas relating to the Feminine and the m/Other.

Luce Irigaray and Julia Kristeva

Ettinger's theory of the matrixial must be distinguished from the writing of Luce Irigaray who posits a Feminine doubling (two lips speaking together), fusion and symbiotic relations. Like Irigaray, Ettinger opposes the phallus as a master signifier but the two theorists differ with respect to how they understand the Feminine. Irigaray posits an auto-erotic or Feminine doubling through her use of two-lips speaking together. Ettinger's formulation of the Feminine does not involve a doubling but rather a borderlinking between the subject and the Other. There is, in other words, a more-than-one and a less-than-one in an asymmetrical borderlinking. For Ettinger, Feminine sexual difference is not auto-erotic but transitive and copoietic. Irigaray's work does not give us a way to understand what Ettinger calls the sub-subjective (the Other in the I) or the trans-subjective (the I in the Other). Irigaray does theorize intrauterine life—as does Ettinger—but again, the formulation differs. As Griselda Pollock (2006) writes in her introduction to Ettinger's *Matrixial Borderspace*, "Luce Irigaray has proposed the placenta to speak about the imaginary and the symbolic of intrauterine life and of the first bodily encounter with the mother" (37). But, as Pollock, notes, Irigaray's formulation attempts to replace the phallus (as predicated upon the penis, male phantasy and desire vis-à-vis women) with another bodily organ particular to female-bodied people. Substitution remains "within a model of presence/absence, severance and loss by castration, and the hallucinatory return of the repressed" (Pollock quoted in Ettinger 2006c, 37). Ettinger's theorization does not aim to replace or to match the phallus but to add a critical supplement to it by way of the matrixial.

The matrix must also be differentiated from Julia Kristeva's writing on the Chora, which also means womb and uterus. Although both the Chora and the Matrix are anchored to maternal encounters, the Chora cannot be symbolized in Kristeva's theory and is relegated to psychotic discourse or to poetic discourse. Ettinger's concern with Kristeva's conceptualization of the Chora is that it reduces birth to psychosis; "giving birth must emerge as psychosis in culture [for Kristeva]" (Ettinger 2000, 204). For Ettinger, this is only true from a phallic perspective that fails to apprehend the subject-as-encounter (or severality) as anything but fusion, symbiosis and/or homogeneity. As explained above, matrixial phenomenon can be symbolized in an expanded Symbolic and is not psychotic. Rather, the matrix is an important component of partial-subjectivity that can be understood in a larger aggregated theoretical formulation involving the matrixial borderspace.

It must also be noted that Kristeva's writing on the Chora focuses on the post-natal while Ettinger's work on the matrixial begins with the prenatal. "The Matrix deals with symbols in relation to prenatal strata of subjectivity, partial objects, differences which do not imply opposition, a-symmetry, more-than-one but not everything, less-than-one but not nothing" (Ettinger 1992, 16). Ettinger is, however, in agreement with the way Kristeva understands the signifying aspects of psychic energy. Specifically the way the body pulsates and trans-connects through corporeal rhythms. Both theorists have also written beautifully on Antigone, sister and daughter of Oedipus in the Theban trilogy (Cavanagh 2017), and make significant contributions to Feminine psychoanalytic ethics.

Another key difference between Ettinger and Kristeva is with respect to their different approaches to the phallus as signifier and to the Lacanian Symbolic. Ettinger's Feminine-matrixial operates alongside but not within the phallic stratum. As already noted, the matrix is not an organ or a metaphor employed to replace the phallus as inaugural signifier. Kristeva's notion of the Feminine and abjection involves an oppositional relation to the phallus and to the Lacanian Symbolic. Hence, her discussion of the intimate revolt in her book by the same name (Oliver, 2002). Kristeva's emphasize on abjection (2024) and revolt (2002) are also distinct from Ettinger's formulation of borderlinking in the matrixial. For Kristeva, abjection is a psychical process through which the child separates from the semiotic body of the maternal figure. More specifically, the child must separate from a bodily interiority associated with the m/other, her drives, phantasies and part-objects.

In her discussion of Ettinger and Kristeva, Griselda Pollock suggests that Kristeva's formulation of the Feminine is "destined either for melancholia (a refusal to negate the mother) or mourning (sublimation through negation of the mother)" (Pollock 2006, 34). While I would not reduce Kristeva's formulation of Feminine revolt to melancholia and mourning—even as these experiences may be features of what Kristeva calls "intimate revolts" and "intimate politics" (2002), there is, as Pollock notes, a difference with respect to the status of the I in pregnancy. Pregnancy is, for Kristeva, a "split identity, a threshold between nature and culture, between biology and language, *with no singularity and no relations to an ethical Other*" (Pollock 2006, 35). Pollock's major critique of Kristeva, as I understand it, is that the pregnant subject is rendered psychotic. She explains, that for Kristeva, the

> *it* is happening…*I* am not there. The *I* cannot think *it* [pregnancy]…the event of the female body is so impossible to think, so impossible to signify, that the woman to whom it happens becomes temporarily dispossessed, psychotic in her own body, unhinged from language itself. (35)

In other words, for Kristeva, the pregnant woman is not a subject; she is unhinged by an *it* that is, for Ettinger, an encounter-event central to an Other axis of sexual difference. For Kristeva, by contrast, pregnancy evokes a kind of psychosis and a paranoid "you" (as *it*) or "me" dynamic. Abjection and revolt in the Kristevian formulation becomes a necessity.

Like Ettinger's writing on the matrixial borderspace, Kristeva's theory of the maternal-infant dyad has made enormous contributions to theorizing a Feminine dimension of experience relevant to the aesthetics, affects, ethics and human reproduction. While Kristeva focuses on the time-space transition from the semiotic to the symbolic, Ettinger focuses on the difference between the Feminine-matrixial sub-stratum and the Symbolic. For Kristeva, the transition to the Symbolic is a gradual and processional time-movement in which the mother takes an active role. She prepares the child for entry into the Symbolic and does so in what Kristeva calls the "thetic" move. The "thetic" time-space of the maternal-infant relation functions like a bridge or threshold between the semiotic and the Symbolic. In Kristeva's model, the child must break the symbiotic bond to become a subject. This separation is understood in terms of castration and abjection, but it should not be forgotten that Kristeva stresses the transitional elements of the developmental sequence whereby the infant becomes a subject. "Castration puts the finishing touches on the process of separation that posits the subject as signifiable, which is to say, separate, always confronted by another" (Kristeva 1986, 47).

Ettinger's critique of the Kristevian formulation is that it requires castration, a cut or radical break from the m/Other. For Kristeva, the child must separate from the mother who is associated with bodily (semiotic) interiority. Ettinger is concerned with the status of the m/Other in the Kristevian formulation and in culture more broadly. Additionally, Ettinger objects to the reduction of pregnancy to psychosis. As explained above, borderlinkings to the m/Other (as first Other) are, from an Ettingerian perspective, important to matrixial subjectivity: the subject-as-several. Furthermore, Ettinger's matrixial-Feminine is about invisible ties and borderlinkings that are un-cognized but central to the human experience. It follows that she is critical of the Kristevian emphasis on abjection which consolidates inner and outer worlds, purity and defilement. As Pollock agrees, the Kristevian abject becomes an alien and it then follows that the Other is "rejected and repulsive" (Pollock 2006, 109). For Ettinger, this is a phallic conceptualization based on castrating splits as opposed to a trans-subjective weave. Ettinger's emphasis is on how best to conceptualize severality, the subject-as-encounter, whereby Kristeva's theory of the subject is more in keeping with the Lacanian approach although she focuses on what we might call the Feminine side.

Another central difference between Ettinger and Kristeva can be observed in the differential emphasis each places upon the emerging I. Ettinger stresses the importance of the I and *non-I* together (as partial-subjectivity), whereas Kristeva stresses the importance of separation between the infant-child-I and the m/Other (castration). For Ettinger, the subject-as-encounter needs their *non-I's* (as Others in the borderlinking), but Kristeva is inclined to worry about fusion and symbiosis in the mother-child dyad. Kristeva is concerned about psychosis in the dyadic relationship, whereas Ettinger contends that pregnancy and after-birth experiences are not psychotic and can be symbolized in an expanded Symbolic. Ettinger refers to pregnancy as a "negated third possibility – an unspeakable, or should we say, evacuated possibility" (Ettinger 2004, 69) in the phallic stratum, but one that can be apprehended in the matrixial. The act of giving birth becomes a void along with the birth-giving mother who becomes, in Ettinger's assessment, the archaic m/Other in the phallic frame. The void is not abject in a Kristevian sense but rather an obscurity.

Kristeva, Julia (2024), has written much about how the archaic mother is understood in the phallic frame. She, like Ettinger, has made tremendous contributions to theorizing the Feminine. Although more scholarly work needs to be done on the differences between Ettinger's approach to the matrixial and Kristeva's formulation of the semiotic, it is fair to say that Kristeva's theorization is, like Ettinger's oeuvre, a critical feminist response to Lacan. While Kristeva seeks to give meaning to the semiotic in the symbolic through, for example, her fiction and theorizations,

Ettinger seeks to show, through her art-theory and writings, the place of the matrixial in the subject as several and wed to Others in difference. Both feminist psychoanalytic theorists and clinicians share a reverence for the Feminine, and there is, in both scholars, a residual Lacanian influence and point of reference. Ettinger and Kristeva both know that something remains unsaid in Lacan's teachings on feminine sexuality. The two theorists should, in my view, also be read together, not because they are the same, but because they are, in different ways, engaging ethical questions about the Feminine. Whether or not one agrees with the limitations of Kristeva's theorizing as illustrated by Pollock and Ettinger, it is important to acknowledge that there are significant differences in the two formulations yet to be fully explored.

Bibliography

Cavanagh, Sheila L. 2017. 'Antigone's Legacy: A Feminist Psychoanalytic of an Other Sexual Difference'. Studies in the Maternal 9(1).

Deleuze, Gilles and Guattari, Felix. 1987. A Thousand Plateaus: Capitalism and Schizophrenia. Translated by Brian Massumi. Continuum Press, London and New York.

Ettinger, Bracha Lichtenberg. 1992. Matrix and Metramorphosis. *Differences: A Journal of Feminist Cultural Studies* 4 (3): 176–209.

Ettinger, Bracha. 1993. Matrix; Halal (A)-Lapsus: Notes on Painting. Museum of Modern Art, 1993.

Ettinger, Bracha. 1996. Metramorphic Borderlinks and Matrixial Borderspace. In *Rethinking Borders*, ed. John C. Welchman. University of Minnesota Press.

Ettinger, Bracha. 1997. The Feminine/Prenatal Weaving in Matrixial Subjectivity-as-Encounter. *Psychoanalytic Dialogues* 7 (3): 367–405.

Ettinger, Bracha. 2000. Bracha Lichtenberg Ettinger: Artworking, 1985–1999 , Artworking, 1985–1999. Ludion: Palais des Beaux-Arts.

Ettinger, Bracha. 2001. Matrixial Gaze and Screen: Other Than Phallic and Beyond the Late Lacan. In *Bodies of Resistance: New Phenomenologies of Politics, Agency, and Culture*, ed. Laura Doyle. Northwestern University Press.

Ettinger, Bracha. 2004. Weaving a Woman Artist With-in the Matrixial Encounter-Event. *Theory, Culture & Society* 21 (1): 69–94.

Ettinger, Bracha Lichtenberg, and Akseli Virtanen. 2005. "Art, Memory, Resistance. A Conversation with Akseli Virtanen." Ephemera: Theory and Politics in Organization 5 (X): 690–702.

Ettinger, Bracha L. 2006a. Fascinance and the Girl-to-M/Other Matrixial Feminine Difference. In *Psychoanalysis and the Image*, ed. Griselda Pollock. Blackwell Publishing Ltd.

Ettinger, Bracha. 2006b. From Proto-Ethical Compassion to Responsibility: Besideness and the Three Primal Mother-Phantasies of Not-Enoughness, Devouring and Abandonment. *Athena* 1 (2): 100–135.

Ettinger, Bracha. 2006c. The Matrixial Borderspace. In *The Matrixial Borderspace*, Theory out of Bounds, vol. 28. University of Minnesota Press.

Ettinger, Bracha Lichtenberg. 2007. Diotima and the Matrixial Transference: Psychoanalytical Encounter-Event as Pregnancy in Beauty. In *Beyond the Threshold: Explorations of Liminality in Literature*, ed. Hein Viljoen and N. Chris. Van der Merwe. Peter Lang.

Ettinger, Bracha Lichtenberg. 2009. "Fragilization and Resistance." Studies in the Maternal 2 (1): 1–31.

Ettinger, Bracha L. 2011. Uncanny Awe, Uncanny Compassion and Matrixial Transjectivity beyond Uncanny Anxiety. *French Literature Series* (Leiden) 38: 1.

Ettinger, Bracha. 2015. *And My Heart Wound Space*. The Wild Pansy Press.

Ettinger, Bracha Lichtenberg. 2016. Laius Complex and Shocks of Maternality: With Franz Kafka and Sylvia Plath. In *Interdisciplinary Handbook of Trauma and Culture*, ed. Haviva Pedaya, David Gurevitz, Yuval Neria, and Yochai Ataria. Springer International Publishing.

Kristeva, Julia. 1986. The Kristeva Reader. Edited by Toril Moi. New York: Columbia Press.

Kristeva, Julia. 2024. *Powers of Horror: An Essay on Abjection*, European Perspectives. Vol. 98. Columbia University Press.

Oliver, Kelly. 2002 The portable kristeva (updated edition)" Columbia University Press, New York.

Pollock, Griselda. 2006. Femininity: Aporia or Sexual Difference? In *The Matrixial Borderspace*, Theory out of Bounds, ed. Bracha Ettinger, vol. 28. University of Minnesota Press.

Pollock, Griselda. 2008. "Beyond Oedipus: Feminist Thought, Psychoanalysis and Mythical Figurations of the Feminine." In Laughing with Medusa: Classical Myth and Feminist Thought, edited by Vanda Zajko and Miriam Leonard, 67–120. Classical Presences. Oxford: Oxford University Press.

Pollock, Griselda. 2013. Art as Transport-Station of Trauma? Haunting Objects in the Works of Bracha Ettinger, Sarah Kofman and Chantal Akerman. In *Representing Auschwitz: At the Margins of Testimony*. Springer.
Zajko, Vanda, and Miriam Leonard, eds. 2006. *Laughing with Medusa: Classical Myth and Feminist Thought*. OUP Oxford.

3

The Other Sexual Difference

This chapter outlines Bracha L. Ettinger's critique of the Freudian-Lacanian field to establish context for her critical feminist supplement to Lacan's theory of sexuation vis-a-vis the Other Sexual Difference (OSD). As discussed in the previous chapter, Ettinger is critical of the way Freud and Lacan neglect intrauterine phantasies along with the womb. Her critique gives rise to a theorization of the OSD, which is, in my assessment, one of the most interesting contributions Ettinger makes to theories of sexuality. The OSD has nothing to do with Oedipal logic or with what Lacan calls sexuation, both of which occur after birth. Brian Massumi, who edited Ettinger's work in *The Matrixial Borderspace*, explains that the matrixial is the "other of the masculine-feminine opposition. Since the matrixial is generative, its otherness to phallic oppositional structure may still be considered a sexual difference. In fact, it is *the* sexual difference, as against the difference between the sexes" (Massumi quoted in Ettinger 2006d, 26). To put this in other terms, the matrixial axis of difference is irreducible to the phallic premise anchoring Lacan's analytic of sexuation. The OSD is not about *having* or *being* the phallus as it is for Lacan but about a non-Oedipal Feminine difference beyond the phallus. The OSD

S. L. Cavanagh, *Bracha L. Ettinger and Jacques Lacan*, The Palgrave Lacan Series,
https://doi.org/10.1007/978-3-032-23293-9_3

does not operate through oppositions, gender identifications, divisions, and phallic cuts because the subject is aware that the m/Other is "alike-non-same" (Ettinger 2006d, 184). It is an axis of difference where the subject-is-several (not One).

While Ettinger distinguishes the OSD from the Other (Feminine) jouissance theorized by Lacan, I contend that there is a relation between the matrixial-Feminine and Lacan's formulation of the Feminine not-all and the Other. Despite Ettinger's critique of Lacan's writings on Feminine sexuality, she is a post-Lacanian feminist scholar whose writings are in dialogue with Lacan. In fact, as I will argue, the OSD is a critical feminist addendum to Lacan's foundational work on the Other Jouissance, the m/Other, the Real, and sexuation. Consider also that Ettinger's terminology and points of reference derive from the Lacanian lexicon. It is therefore important to ground her feminist supplement in Lacanian theory. In so doing, I elucidate what is unique and different about the Ettingerian approach. I introduce the OSD through Ettinger's writings on the matrixial gaze and in relation to what she calls pre-birth incest (as distinct from after-birth incest); a form of incest that is not only essential to life but to the matrixial borderspace. But let us begin by considering the place of intrauterine phantasies in Freudian and Lacanian psychoanalysis to better understand and evaluate Ettinger's claim that pre-birth experiences are submerged in their writings.

Intrauterine Fantasies

Psychoanalysis usually pays tribute to the boy as son and to the man as father while the girl as daughter and the woman as mother languish in Ettinger's assessment. She contends that the obstacle to understanding the Feminine dimension of experience is grounded in a long-standing failure to give the pre-birth encounter-event between the mother-to-be and the subject-to-be analytic attention. In her view, Freud and Lacan pay insufficient attention to intrauterine experience or related phantasies involving the mother as first Other. While Freud listened to his male patients talk about womb-envy and reflects upon pre-birth phantasies, these elements of experience are not only undertheorized in Ettinger's assessment, but understood from the perspective of the man who is Oedipal. Pre-birth experiences and intrauterine phantasies are referred to in Freud, but they receive significantly less attention than those elements of experience associated with the boy's after-birth experience of the castration complex.

While Freud does acknowledge the place of the womb in the sexual curiosities of young children, Ettinger claims that he thought it necessary to deny them. She reasons that Freud thought it necessary for the (boy) child to deny the womb in the service of his (healthy) narcissism and masculine identification. In other words, Freud believed that it was necessary to deny the womb and the mysteries associated with childbirth to support male narcissism and the concordant denial of Feminine sexual difference. As Ettinger explains:

> Freud did not deny the denial of the womb nor its implications. On the contrary. He insisted on the necessity of such a denial, measured by the enormity of what is at stake for males. He considers the penis the central support of "the child's" narcissism (what child, we may ask – male or female?) and the "enigma of the sphinx: where do children come from?" as central for sexual development of the male child." (2006d, 174)

Freud concludes that it was natural to deny and displace knowledge relating to the sexual specificity of reproduction. He bases this conclusion, in part, on his analysis of anal birth fantasies in his adult-male-clients. In Ettinger's reading of Freud, the father of psychoanalysis thought that the negation of the womb was essential to Oedipal development for boys-becoming-man. Men deny the corpo-Real[1] sexual difference of the woman-becoming-mother by believing that they too could give birth. In the Freudian interpretation, as Ettinger understands it, the male-boy cannot tolerate the narcissistic blow to his ego by acknowledging that he lacks something as significant as the womb.

Ettinger also questions the premise that *Mutterliebsphantasie*—maternal womb/intrauterine phantasies—are necessarily frightening as Freud

---

[1] Corpo-reality (unlike corporeality) is mediated by phantasy, desire, affective-linkages to Others (as *non-I*'s), aesthetics and the unique composition of any given matrixial webbing.

suggests in his writing on the uncanny [*Das Unheimliche*].[2] Freud's theorization of the uncanny is largely about the vaginal origins of birth, what is felt to be intimate and foreign, repressed but emergent in everyday experience, much like *déjè vu*. Lacan explains that the "feeling of d *déjè vu* comes to meet the erratic hallucination, that it is the imaginary echo which arises as a response to a point of reality that belongs to the limit where it has been excised from the symbolic" (Lacan 2006b, 326). What is evident in Lacan's theorization of the imaginary echo and the limit is, for Ettinger, the body-memory of the womb in need of analytic attention. Indeed, we may read Ettinger's theorization of the matrixial borderspace as an extensive mapping of what has been excised from the Symbolic: specifically, a Feminine dimension of experience where the birth-giving mother is essential. In Ettinger's careful reading of Freud, she reasons that intrauterine phantasies become frightening only when repressed and subject to castration anxiety in the phallic axis of difference (the Lacanian Symbolic as distinct from what Ettinger calls the matrixial-Feminine sub-Symbolic). Noting that children often ask questions about where babies come from before they ask questions about what it means to be a man or a woman, Ettinger establishes that that differences between the child-subject and the mother predates sexual difference (as difference between the sexes).

What all children first seek to understand is where they came from. What Freud refers to as the child's sexual research into the mysteries of birth, begins with a non-genital sexual interest in the mother. What Freud refers to as intrauterine fantasies are foundational to the OSD. While the early years of life are, as Freud argues, unremembered but unconsciously inscribed, for Ettinger, they give phenomenological and phantasmatic form to the OSD. But more than this, the pre-birth experiences of the subject tethered to the becoming-mother are unconsciously registered and give form to an-Other dimension of subjectivity. This is, in the Ettingerian paradigm, the subject-as-several (or severality). The matrixial subject is borderlinked to their Others (or *non-I*'s) in matrixial webs. This borderlinking is, as already noted, central to the

[2] See: Sigmund, Freud, and McLintock David. "The uncanny." *The Standard Edition of the Complete Psychological Works of Sigmund Freud* 17 (1919): 1917–1919.

OSD where individuals do not exist without Others. Ettinger also refers to the severality of the subject to underscore the way we are borderlinked to Others, whom she also calls our *non-Is*. A *non-I* is a discerning element that does not involve separation (or castration) but togetherness with-in-difference.

In Ettinger's feminist critique, denial of the womb is accompanied by male-masculine appropriation: "In psychoanalysis, the phantasy of the maternal womb is *excluded by inclusion* within the "castration" phantasy! "Castration," which is a sexual notion even though the "phallus" is considered neutral, is the prototype of *any* separation from the bodily and archaic partial dimension, of any loss and absence that leads to an inscription in the Symbolic" (Ettinger 2006d, 47). By denying the sexual and reproductive specificity of the birth-giving mother and the Feminine axis of difference more generally, Ettinger contends that Freud elevates the boy-as-future-man to a universal standard and point of reference. "For Freud, the male's bodily specificity—the penis—is regarded as the *only* index for sex difference for *both* sexes; the sexuality of girls is fundamentally male, and the libido has only one essence" (95). Libido is thus masculine and, as Freud writes, "little girls" are "little boys." Lacan does not fare much better in Ettinger's assessment. She argues that the womb is, for Lacan, "foreclosed, perhaps logically excluded, by inclusion in the "castration" prototype that alone informs and structures all objects as lacking, beginning with the mother-object" (175). As a result, Ettinger concludes that psychoanalysts prioritize the phantasy of one-ness, the "sovereign One, the phallic Symbolic" (54).

By neglecting matrixial elements of experience in psychoanalysis and culture at large, we do a disservice to the Feminine dimension of experience. Moreover, Ettinger claims that the male-boy-man appropriates the gestational and birth-giving capacities of the mother and transfers them onto the man in what she calls the genius-male-hero complex. "Thus, the denial that allows for secretive and buried appropriation of maternal gestation, begetting, birth-giving, and love in the service of father-son relations creates the Genius-Hero myth on the sacrifice of the eliminated and evaporated archaic Woman-m/Other" (175). For Ettinger, the neglect or pathologization of the Feminine dimension of experience, coupled with gestational appropriation, stems from a neglect of the Feminine dimension of experience she observes in Freud and Lacan.

Ettinger contends that the Feminine dimension of experience and everything bodily relating to it is subsumed into the Oedipal-castration model by Freud and later by Lacan in his formulation of the (phallic) Symbolic. As many feminist psychoanalysts critical of the way the mother is neglected, blamed, or pathologized in the psychoanalytic literature might agree, there is, as Ettinger argues, a discourse, desire, and aesthetic particular to the maternal-Feminine missing in Freudian and Lacanian theory. As she explains, "Any feminine alterity beyond the phallus can't be inscribed: whatever does not obey phallic principles can't be recognized; and anything recognized via the symbolic system is already phallic" (Ettinger 1997, 375). But does Lacan actually foreclose on the Feminine dimension of experience as Ettinger contends or, is it, perhaps, more accurate to say that his elaboration of the Feminine is partial and, in his view, best left to female psychoanalysts whom he calls out for not having given their all to the removal of secrets relating to the Other jouissance? I ask this not to be an apologist for Lacan (or even Freud), but because there are, in my feminist reading, matrixial seeds planted in Lacan's teachings.

Lacan and the Woman

Lacanian readers may be quick to take issue with Ettinger's premise that the m/Other is not a central figure in his writings. Moreover, Lacanians may reasonably counter that there is a Woman (who does not exist) in Lacanian theory and that she should not be mistaken for actual women who do exist. Lacanian theory is not meant to be sexist or neglectful of the Feminine dimension of experience. To the contrary, it is meant to elucidate a logic whereby the Woman is not all subject to the phallic signifier. In other words, there is something, on the Feminine side, that allows women to experience an Other (non-phallic) jouissance that can, from the perspective of enjoyment, be advantageous.

In more precise Lacanian terms, the Lacanian Woman is not-all subject to the phallic premise and this is what enables her to experience an

Other (Feminine) jouissance. Although there is a difference between the Woman and the m/Other in the Lacanian account, it cannot be said that he underestimates the m/Other in his writings although he may be faulted for having failed to say as much about the maternal function as he does the paternal function. Consider that Lacan writes about *lalangue* (combining *langue* and *la*), which is, in effect, the language of the mother (and not delimited by the rules of language) and about the law of the mother (Morel 2018). In *Seminar IV* on the object relation, Lacan refers to the "the (Real) almightiness of the mother" (2020, 185–186) and in his discussion of *object a* (a non-object cause of desire), he explains that she is the ultimate *Thing* (*das Ding*) around which desire pivots. While Ettinger reads this "Thing" as sexist and objectifying, it is, for Lacan, a central and important residue of what remains from a phallic (signifying) cut from the m/Other.

Lacan believes that our entry into the Symbolic is not via the m/Other but through the signifier.[3] In other words, we come into existence through a castrating word-like cut. The trouble with this formulation is that it does not allow for those elements of human experience that are not delimited by the word-image. Ettinger contends that theories of subjectivity must take account of those aspects of human experience that are in excess of the Symbolic. More to the Ettingerian point, there is a Feminine pre-discursive dimension before the signifier that Lacan neglects in his theory of the subject. Ettinger refers to Félix Guattari, who notes, the "linguistic signifier in no way encloses all of the components combining to produce subjectivity" (Ettinger 2002, 244).

Equally, Ettinger is critical of the threat Lacan supposes the m/Other poses to the child. For her, this smacks of sexism. Lacan emphasizes the importance of the paternal function and the way it must interdict the desire of the m/Other. The (Real) almightiness of the mother (Lacan 2020, pp. 185–186) must be neutralized in Lacan's considered opinion by a phallic cut (signifier) for the benefit of the child. In his discussion of the object relation in *Seminar IV*, Lacan refers to the "unfulfilled and

[3] The Lacanian reliance upon language has been critiqued by analysts like Dider Anzieu (1989). Others, like Paul Schilder (2013 [1950]), who have gone on to develop psychoanalytically informed theories of the postural model of the body are also critical of the privileged position given to language in Lacanian psychoanalysis.

unsatisfied mother ... [who] is in search of what she can devour, *quaerens quem devoret*" (187). He also insists that his students understand the power of the mother, the way imaginary objects are bound to the maternal body, and the way the "mother constitutes a virtual field of symbolic annihilation, from which each of the objects to come will in turn draw their symbolic value" (178). The m/Other is what Lacan believes "structures [the] man's unconscious," she is the "terminal point, the abolition of the whole world of demand" (Lacan 1992, p. 68).

Lacan and Ettinger might agree that the position and function of the m/Other is central. But Ettinger disagrees with the risks posed by the m/Other in the Lacanian frame. Moreover, she takes issue with the way the m/Other needs to be interdicted by the paternal function. As I will discuss in the next chapter, Ettinger is highly critical of the way the Woman is reduced to *object a* (*das Ding*) in Lacan's theory, a non-object cause of desire for the boy-man. Additionally, Lacan may be said to discount an axis of desire related to being in relation to Others and otherness that Ettinger theorizes through her discussion of the matrixial sinthome (Cavanagh 2016) (an older word for symptom central to the later work of Lacan). If it is true that Lacan eclipses or, at least, leaves undertheorized a dimension of experience relating to what Ettinger calls the matrixial-Feminine, this has understudied implications for girls and women (trans and cisgender) as I discuss in the following chapters focused on Tiresias, Dora, Marguerite Duras, and Antigone.

In Ettinger's account, the bodily specificity of the m/Other including her reproductive capacity, Real and imagined, is important. Given the centrality of sexual positioning in Lacan's teachings, it is curious that he does not say more about who the m/Other is for the girl as distinct from who she is for the boy. For Lacan, there are two ways of being in relation to the phallic premise: masculine (all subject to the phallic premise); and Feminine (not-all subject to the phallic premise). But if there is a sexual difference between Feminine and masculine subjects in Lacan's teachings (the only two choices available for sexuated subjects), why does he sideline the difference sexuation makes to our divergent relations to the m/Other as object cause of desire, as agent of demand and jouissance?

The answer is not evident or straightforward in Lacan's teachings. But in Ettinger's view, Lacan's writings on the Woman and the m/Other are elaborated from the "man's side." In other words, Lacan gives us a way to understand the discourse, desire, affect and aesthetics of the Feminine and the m/Other from the perspective of the masculine dimension of experience, but not from the Feminine dimension of experience which has a unique relevance to the lives of girls and women.

In the chapters to follow, I will analyze what Ettinger refers to as matrixial complexes in the case of Dora (Freud's canonical case of female hysteria), Lol Stein (in Margarite Duras's novel), and in Antigone (of the Sophocles trilogy), but let us, in this chapter, concentrate our focus on the Ettingerian critique of Freud and Lacan while, also, introducing her analytic of the OSD. For Ettinger, there are clinical problems with the appropriation of the Feminine into the Oedipal-castration model. Her feminist conclusion is that psychoanalysis, as envisioned from the perspective of Oedipus, is not equally salient to natal male and natal female subjects (regardless of gender identity, trans- and cisgender): it is specific to the "male body, to its pleasures and pains and to the phantasies attached to it" (Ettinger 2006d, 179). Much like castration anxiety emerges for the boy, what Ettinger calls matrixial complexes (or intrauterine complexes) cause anxiety for the girl especially, but also for the boy, when repressed and subject to negation. Denial of the m/Other in psychoanalysis and in culture more broadly effects both girls and boys (regardless of gender identity), but it has a uniquely damaging effect upon the cisgender girl-becoming-woman (and potential future mother) due to the way the cisgender girl-child's sexual morphology more closely resembles the mother's body. In order to correct what Ettinger views as a phallic oversight in Lacan's teachings, she develops a formulation of the OSD relevant to the matrixial borderspace.

The Other Sexual Difference

Through her analytic of the OSD (and her art-practice), Ettinger seeks to inscribe both the Woman and the sexual rapport, which, for her, exists in the OSD, and restore both to sense if not to direct signification. This is to say that in the OSD, there is, for Ettinger, a sexual rapport on the Feminine side. Referring to the OSD, Ettinger writes "if we want to claim a supplementary unconscious zone in subjectivity, a different experience is not enough. Other structures, mechanisms, and functions have to be looked for, as well as a different kind of inscription for transferring events into subjectivity" (Ettinger 1997, 374–375). To put this in other terms, the OSD is Ettinger's answer to the phallic signifier and to phallic logic where, in Lacan, the Woman does not exist. We may understand the OSD as that which is submerged in Lacanian psychoanalysis but nevertheless struggles to make itself known. As Ettinger explains, it "struggles to open up, a difference that has nothing to do with Oedipal man/woman difference, but which accompanies and subtends it" (2006a, 89). The OSD does not operate according to the signifiers of concern to Lacan but through the language of the body. Ettinger refers to the "language of bodily signs…[and to] the language of affective channelings, the language of transference that 'speaks' with its sensations and affectations among subjects that co-emerge or co-fade in a matrixial alliance" (2006d, 184).

The OSD is based upon a prenatal difference or a "uterine differential relation" (Neill 2008, 330). It is predicated upon non-linguistic elements of experience that are unconscious and harken back to bodily experiences involving the primal scene of birth and the mother-Other/other Other's body, experiences that Ettinger does not view to be essential but matrixial (and thus irreducible to the organ and to the image).

Although not all females can or desire to give birth, Ettinger bases her theory of the OSD, or at least part of it, on the capacity, imagined and Real, of female reproduction. While "Woman" in Ettingerian theory does not symbolize natal female sex but a complex borderlinking, female corpo-Reality signifies something of importance to psychical experience. In the Ettingerian frame, sex (or gender) neutrality in contemporary culture is not about inclusion but a negation of female sexual morphology and its relation to the reproductive function (Real and imagined). Ettinger elaborates:

> I believe that to avoid dealing with any aspect that touches on the female body and bodily experience, to avoid the conceptual potentiality that can be abstracted from the female body or has consequences with regard to it and its history – the agglomeration of its traumatic or pleasurable

> experiences, its potentiality, the phantasies that link to its inscriptions – I believe that this amounts to an unconditional surrender to the dominant, seemingly neutral, symbolic filter that censures both women and men and molds them in its phallic frame. (2006d, 179–180)

While reproductive capacity matters in Ettingerian theory, her reference to body parts, like the womb, is mediated by phantasy, desire, trauma, and jouissance particular to the OSD. As such, it would be a mistake to assume that the signifier "womb" is (only) a material organ and not, also, a signifying apparatus. Ettinger intends "womb" to stand for a psychic capacity for sharability and borderlinking. It is *not* to be taken as a discrete organ per se. Ettinger explains:

> The male sexual organ is a support for the conceptualization of the phallic-Oedipal field with its castration complex, but the phallus [in Lacan] is not to be identified with the penis. Similarly, the womb, fetus, pregnancy, and gestation, as corpo-Realities and image, are supports for a matrixial field of theorization; likewise, the idea of the matrix should not be identified with the womb, nor Woman with Mother. (2006d, 183)

What Ettinger attempts to make clear is that the natal sex specificity of the body is a metaphorical grounding for both phallic and matrixial sexual differences. In effect, she supplants Lacan's equation "Phallus = Symbol" with "Phallus + Matrixial (+ possibly other concepts) = Symbol" (Ettinger 1992, 190). But it can be argued that she repeats an essentialist metonymy by linking the idea of the womb to the female body; much like Lacan may be said to establish a metonymy by linking the phallus to masculine experience. While Ettinger, like Lacan, is correct to underscore the Real, Symbolic, and Imaginary dimensions of the matrixial and phallic-Oedipal fields, the question of sexual morphology and reproductive differences, however we might agree to understand them, are relevant to both theoretical formations.

This is why Ettinger argues, for instance, that phantasies of weaning must not be folded into the Freudian castration complex (although they may be co-existent). Matrixial complexes involve bodily affects (that we may liken to Lacan's part-objects and traces) "informed by *touching*, *hearing*, *voice*, and *moving*, not plainly connected with particular erogenetic areas, nor uniquely connected with bodily orifices…[but] composed by linking and relating" (Ettinger 2006d, 48). These borderlinkings at the origin of life give way to the OSD where one cannot be without an m/Other. The OSD may be non-linguistic but "its traces would be engraved in an unconscious sphere that is not equivalent to the repressed chain of signifiers" (Ettinger 1997, 376) in the Lacanian frame. We might understand Ettinger's affective trace inscriptions of jouissance in terms of Lacan's markers, or what he calls invasive signifiers, imprinted on the subject's body by the Other.

In Ettinger's theorization, reproductive capacity matters, as does sexual morphology, but how it matters for the girl as distinct from the boy is not absolute. For Ettinger, the female body comes with an imprint of an enigma of an "encounter – between *I* and *non-I* in coemergence" (2007, 127). She admits that the male body also comes with an imprint of an enigmatic encounter with the m/Other, but what it means for the boy-son is yet to be worked out. For all becoming-subjects regardless of sexual morphology, the first *non-I* is the mother-to-be experienced by the subject-to-be through joint sensations and affective links in utero. As Ettinger explains, the specificity of the prenatal encounter inscribes a Real (unsignifiable) trace-like link between the becoming-subject and the m/Other where her desire, trauma and jouissance is transferred. The matrixial is not delimited by the signifier (as is the Lacanian Symbolic), but by an unconscious borderspace of co-emergence and co-fading in the Feminine matrixial.

In this other sphere, we can apprehend the presence of Others who are not absolute others. They are, for Ettinger, *non-I*'s tethered in a trans-subjective borderspace that she compares to a web or textured plait. While Lacan refers to language as a web, a "mesh of signifiers" (Lacan 1997, Seminar III), Ettinger's matrixial web is not about signifiers but rather affective and aesthetic traces that recall the m/Other's body. Neither fused nor rejected, the *I* and the *non-I* enable subjectification through/in encounter events in the matrixial borderspace. Ettinger explains that the matrix is an "unconscious borderspace" that remembers female bodily specificity but is not based on "essence, identity, or negation" (1997, 368). The OSD is predicated upon a "shareable dimension of subjectivity" where both *I* and *non-I* "co-emerge and co-inhabit a joint space" (Ettinger 2007, 65) that is matrixial. Ettinger refers to the *non-I* as a site of transmission to be distinguished from an Other as individual-subject. The co-emergence and co-inhabiting are enabled by a border-linking that is Real, phantasmatic, and *jouissant*. The borderlinking is an encounter-event in the Real (a psychic register that cannot be signified) at the basis of Feminine sexual difference. It is felt "in/by the Real" (Ettinger 1997, 401). The Other (Feminine) sexual difference "produces for men and women a different, non-Oedipal sublimation where, in the search for *non-I*(s), the *jouissance* is of the borderlinking itself" (Ettinger 2001, 110).

The matrixial is moored by a primordial heterogeneity, a non-unified Feminine zone in all subjects that precedes the law, the Lacanian Symbolic, and the signifier. Ettinger contends that matrixial sexual difference is developmentally *before* phallic sexual difference but does not end with Oedipalization or sexuation. Nor is it subsumed by these phallic, developmental, and structural axis of difference. In Ettinger's formulation, Feminine sexual difference emerges before, during and after Oedipalization. The matrixial is not Feminine in the phallic sense of the term because it is an originary and primordial difference that predates sexuation and the Oediapl stage. The matrixial is "modeled on intimate sharing in *jouissance,* trauma, and phantasy in the feminine/prebirth sphere, and the womb stands for a psychic capacity for sharability created in the borderlinking to a female body" (Ettinger 2006d, 181). In other words, the feminine matrixial upsets the belief in what Ettinger calls the "*subjectivity supported by a One* (separate of fused)" (Ettinger 2006d, 87). We may say (although Ettinger does not) that the Man does not exist (as One) in the matrixial sub-Symbolic.

The Other axis of sexual difference is primary and foundational to the subject. In the OSD, there is a viable and essential place for the Woman (as a complex borderlinking and condition of co-emergence), the m/Other, and the Feminine. Contra Lacan, Ettinger contends that the Woman can be represented from the Feminine side. She concedes that the Woman may be not-all there in the Symbolic anchored to the phallic premise in the Lacanian equation, but she, nevertheless, exists and must be signified. In Ettinger's terms, the Woman has a borderline presence that can be apprehended in an expanded sub-Symbolic (which I will discuss below). Her theory of the matrixial is intended to conjure up the Woman who is there and not there in Lacan.

The question of the OSD is initially posed to a m/Other (or primary caregiver). More specifically, it is a "sex difference linked to female bodily specificity [that] produces for the man and the woman an-other subjective and objective sphere…[And] the woman is confined neither to one-body nor to either-sex boundaries" (Ettinger 2006d, 95). The matrixial offers us a passage to the Real through visual and aesthetic fields where our *non-I*'s converge, co-mingle, and co-exist. Ettinger hypothesizes that the Feminine Symbolic (occluded by the phallic Symbolic stratum) touches upon the Real and forges a link (in the phallic Symbolic stratum) to a female body schemata (Real and imagined). Because female "body schema are not inscribed in the Symbolic" (Ettinger 1992), it is important to be attentive to non-discursive resonant vibrations and nonconscious memories of female sex specific corporeality. Un-cognized memories of the early mother-to-be/late fetal sexual relations leave trace inscriptions, mediate affects, and produces internal sensations that operate in the matrixial substratum.

Ettinger demonstrates how the OSD is analyzable via traces, aesthetic objects, *a-links* (as distinct from the Lacanian a-object), and encounter-events in what she calls matrixial webs. Matrixial encounter-events are attuned to co-affective linkages (which she calls *a-links*), affective traces and aesthetics between partial-subjects who co-emerge, mutate, and change in assemblage-like relations. These relations harken back to un-remembered time in utero. The affective resonances between the becoming-subject and the becoming-mother are Real (beyond symbolization), affective, and involve an aesthetic particular to the Feminine-matrixial.

In the prenatal encounter, there is, for Ettinger, a non-phallic sexual difference involving the natal female body that is Real (in Lacanian terms[4]). While for Lacan the Real body is fragmented before the mirror-

[4] The Lacanian Real body is distinct from the Imaginary body (where the ego functions). The Real body lacks coherence, undermines identity, and is fragmented (as in the *corps morcelé*). It is also a body that is transitive, thereby obfuscating differences between the self-subject and the Other.

stage (and we are haunted by the gaze of the Other who intercepts us), the matrixial gaze re-installs the Feminine *as* a borderlinking. Lacan famously says that we enter the world as *hommelettes* (scrambled subjects); corporeal disorganization involving subjective dislocation, feelings and phantasies of evisceration, dismemberment, castration, and so forth are Real parts of the human bodily experience. But from a matrixial angle, this scrambled subject is a borderlinking that can be discerned in the sub-Symbolic.

The Sub-Symbolic

In order to theorize Real bodily experience relating to the OSD, Ettinger supplements the Lacanian Symbolic with what she calls the sub-Symbolic. Her critical supplement is inspired by what she identifies as the Freudian position that the prenatal is without sense, a position she also finds in Lacan's views on psychoanalytic practice. Lacan issues a warning to his students that "whosoever dares deal with the matter of the prenatal could not be called a psychoanalyst and would have to be excommunicated" (Ettinger 2006d, 181). Ettinger is equally critical of how

gestation and elements of Feminine experience are associated with psychosis or, at least, with what lacks sense in the Lacanian frame. In her critical assessment of Lacan's failure to theorize gestation, Ettinger says:

> Because women have the emotional capacity to negotiate the unknown Other-with-in during pregnancy without psychosis, something in a Symbolic wider than the phallic-Symbolic allows them some access to this beyond/before in the matrixial stratum, even if the way it conveys meaning is yet to be discovered/invented. (1997, 388)

In order to make sense of pregnancy (as distinct from psychosis), Ettinger posits a sub-Symbolic (which she also refers to in more general terms as the matrixial). The matrixial sub-Symbolic registers that which exceeds the word-image (signifier) and cannot be contained by it. It apprehends elements of the Feminine experience, including reproduction, that, in Lacanian terms, are Real (unsignifiable). Another way to think about the matrixial sub-Symbolic, from the perspective of Lacan, is to say that it provides an organizing symbolic structure for human experiences that are not-all subject to the (phallic) signifier. It operates for everyone, regardless of sexual positioning, but is anchored by the primary experience of gestation involving the m/Other.

The matrixial sub-Symbolic dimension is outside the tentacles of the organ and image. It must be noted that Ettinger is more likely to refer to the "non-conscious" as opposed to the "unconscious" because the former, unlike the latter (in Lacanian parlance), is not an assemblage of repressed signifiers. For Lacan, the "unconscious is the Other's discourse" (Lacan 2006d),[5] but for Ettinger, there is an amnesiac component to psychical life that has a borderline presence. Rather than metaphor and metonymy, Ettinger writes about amnesia—which is not forgotten or repressed.

Ettinger's theorization of the matrixial sub-Symbolic exists alongside the Lacanian Symbolic but is not a substitute for it. There is, for her, a phallic and matrixial dimension to the Symbolic that is not complimentary so much as it is supplementary: the former dimension involving "one-ness, totality, sameness, and Oedipal, symbolic castration" (Ettinger 1992, 2 and 193), the latter involving the Feminine as an "otherness beyond the phallus" (2). This is to say that the Symbolic is Oedipal and thus predicated upon an idea of the individual-One (man), while the sub-Symbolic is non-Oedipal and transitive (involving the *I* and *non-I*'s in a matrixial covenant). Ettinger stresses the way the sub-Symbolic (which is Real) operates alongside but is irreducible to the Lacanian Symbolic (based on language, the Law, and the phallic signifier). The Lacanian Symbolic is phallic because speech, language and discourse are structured by the phallic premise and, in Ettinger's view, dependent upon oppositions, binary thinking dependent on being/not-being all (1997, 371).

But having said this, Ettinger acknowledges that Lacan knows about the "*beyond-the-phallus* feminine sphere" (374) and that, for women, there is what he calls a "radical difference of that which happens on the other side" (quoted in Ettinger 1997, 374). Lacan attempts to get at this other side through the signifier, which, for him, is not purely linguistic.

---

[5] For Lacan 'I' is an-Other.

In the Lacanian frame, subjectivity is about the interdictions of the signifier. In fact, the signifier has a hooking function that involves the Other. In, for example, Lacan's critique of Daniel Lagache's discussion of psychoanalysis and personality structure (1960), he acknowledges the central importance of the "signifiers…linked in a discourse" (Lacan 2006a, 547) that emerge from the Other. For Lacan the desire of the Other, regardless of parentage, casts a determinative die, or mark, upon the subject. The "attributes" or "rudiments" of existence that Lacan focuses on in his critique of Lagache's presentation *are not autonomous*. There is, in other words, an Other which, during gestation is the becoming-mother. What Lagache refers to as "primal differentiation" in his presentation neglects, in Lacan's view, not only the signifying structure but also a Real object-relation. "To my mind, the fact of primal differentiation leaves in abeyance its properly signifying use, on which the advent of the subject depends. To define this primal differentiation in itself, I would say that it is an object-relation *in the real*" (548).

What Lacan refers to as an object-relation in the Real resonates with and may, in fact, be an early iteration of the OSD. It should also be noted that Lacan is critical of the way Lagache refers to the "symbiotic relationship" the child allegedly has with the mother and asks, sardonically, if "they constitute a lichen?" (548). Equally, he takes issue with the presumption that there is symmetry between the child and the Other (parent). Just as Ettinger theorizes the relationship between the subject-to-be and the mother-to-be as asymmetrical and non-symbiotic in the matrixial borderspace, Lacan suggests that what developmental psychologists call maturation involves an emergence from and in a discourse anticipating the child's being. "In my view, the subject has to arise from the given state of the signifiers that cover him [*le recouvrent*] in an Other which is their transcendental locus" (549).

While Lacan gestures to what we might call a "beyond-the-phallus feminine sphere," it is too oblique for Ettinger. She says that he does not theoretically develop this "psychic sphere were supplementary sexual difference might exist" (Ettinger 1997, 375). Moreover, there is a form of relating that predates the signifier. While this may be true, Lacan does concede that there is a jouissance of the body that is not altogether linguistic. But the Imaginary register, like the Symbolic and the Real, are only analyzable via discourse in Lacan's estimate. Preverbal communication does not interest him and is only helpful to the extent that it leads the analyst to a better understanding of the symptom and its linguistic structure. Lacan is resigned to the view that not everything sexual is analyzable and that the analyst must stay focused upon the discourse of the patient. What may be felt and lived in excess of the word as signifier is not, clinically speaking, relevant because it cannot be, as Lacan claims, the focus of analytic interpretation.

Ettinger, by contrast, believes that the OSD is relevant to psychoanalysis and to culture at large. But despite this difference, the Feminine sub-Symbolic postulated by Ettinger corresponds, in my view, to Lacan's theorization of the pre-subjective and the pre-symbolic position of the not-yet-speaking subject. For Ettinger, the matrixial sub-Symbolic is not something we move through as we enter the Symbolic as speaking subjects. We exist in the matrixial sub-Symbolic before, during, and after the phallic order of difference. Lacan's writing on *lalangue* (relating to the mother tongue) where the signifier takes on a relation to a jouissance of the body as distinct from communication is also resonate with Ettinger's formulation of the sub-Symbolic which is moored by the m/Other. As already outlined, Ettinger formulates a theory of the sub-Symbolic to account not only for what she calls "beyond-the-phallus experiences" (2006d, 63), but to establish a groundwork for the OSD, which predates the signifier. From the perspective of the OSD we can apprehend a "matrixial stratum of subjectivization" (64) that is other to an axis of difference arbitrated by the foundational phallic signifier. This stratum of subjectivization involves traumas and phantasies relating to the m/Other. It also involves a mode of subjectivization that is a "One-less, between-the-several" (64) relational zone. Ettinger explains:

> I have termed this layer the matrixial stratum of subjectivization, proposing a matrixial subjectivity-as-encounter as a beyond-the-phallus feminine field related (in both men and women) to plural, partial, and shared unconscious, trauma, phantasy, and desire having imaginary and symbolic impact (and not only an ex-istence in the Real). (2006d, 64)

Ettinger's formulation of the matrixial stratum is what enables her to theorize sub-symbolic interconnectivity, a Feminine dimension of experience that Lacan was unable to elucidate from the Feminine side. As Ettinger explains, the OSD "produces for the man and the woman another subjective and objective sphere" (95): the matrixial stratum or sub-Symbolic. The matrixial sub-Symbolic is a subjectivizing and not regressive. In this way, Ettinger distinguishes the sub-Symbolic from the Kristevian pre-symbolic (predicated upon fusion and symbiosis). "Subsymbolic tunings that do not function on the level of distinct units of signification create meanings that open up the boundaries of culture" (89).

The matrixial sub-Symbolic offers us a passage to the Real through visual and aesthetic fields where our *non-I*'s converge, co-mingle and co-exist. Not only does Ettinger posit an Other symbolic in the Feminine dimension (to which we all participate on an unconscious level), but she says that the matrixial—which operates in this aesthetic landscape—is another supplementary route to the Symbolic. In other words, we not only enter the Symbolic (and thus become subjects) through Oedipalization and through the signifier, but also by matrixial co-affectivity. The Feminine Symbolic touches upon the Real and forges a link to female body schemata. Because female "body schema are not inscribed in the Symbolic" (Ettinger 1992), it is important to be attentive to non-discursive resonant vibrations and nonconscious memories of female sex specific corporeality. Ettinger writes:

> I take the feminine/prenatal meeting as a model for relations and processes of change and exchange in which the *non-I* is unknown to the *I* (or rather uncognized: known by a noncognitive process), but not an intruder. Rather, the *non-I* is a *partner-in-difference* of the *I*. The *late* intrauterine encounter represents, reflects and provides meaning to internal and external realities related to non-Oedipal sexual difference viewed through the prism of the feminine *beyond-the –phallus*. (Ettinger 2006d, 64–65)

Ettinger further suggests that each of us stores archaic traces of this pre-birth encounter-event. This pre-birth encounter is, for her, a condition involving sub-symbolic connectivity. The traces are laced by trauma and phantasy and thus touch upon desire. "They are remembered without being recollected and are revealed in a phantasm saturated with imprints of the trauma of a partial and shared subjectivity" (Ettinger 2001, 109). Traces of these imprints circulate "by affects and by waves" (109), which Ettinger calls erotic antennae of the psyche and these traces are unconscious.

Experiences in utero resonate and vibrate throughout the course of one's life. They are, as Ettinger tells us, aesthetic experiences in excess of the word-image concerning the (phallic) Symbolic. Ettinger notes that these tunings are both stains on the Imaginary and holes in the Real (Ettinger 2006d, 89). She also theorizes psychic transmission and receptivity which are, for Ettinger, filled with "meaning-revelation/production capacities, beyond meanings of being/non-being, having/not having [that are] shareable in phantasy and art" (88). These trace-like weaves of transmission and receptivity comprise un-thought events, traumas, and phantasies that are trans-generational. Of course, we should not presume that these traces are confined to recognizable familial units. They circulate and are reconfigured in community and culture more generally through erotic antennae or "eroticized aerials" (88).

Ettinger's sub-Symbolic enables us to better apprehend psychic experiences, affect, and sensorium in excess of the signifier. The sub-Symbolic is accessible through a matrixial filter. It allows us to create meaning from resonant and apparition-like traces in the trans-subjective and sub-subjective dimensions. The Ettingerian sub-Symbolic is attuned to what lies between and with-in the cut of the signifier. It apprehends gaps between the flesh (of the body) and the word(s) used to not only signify but constitute the body. Borders are, in the sub-Symbolic, not absolute borders, binaries, or splits and cuts. They are generative spaces of co-emergence, hybrid zones of cross-pollination, apparitions on the cusp of the visible and so forth. The sub-Symbolic is in-tune to affective transmissions in the matrixial borderspace that are subjectifying, not psychotic.

Rather than conceiving of the Feminine position as a horizon hovering dangerously close to psychosis (or a point beyond a Symbolic barrier), it is, as Ettinger contends, necessary to conceptualize a transgressive incestuous borderlinking in the matrixial that enables subjectivity-as-encounter.

Incest and the Matrixial

Ettinger contends that the phantasy of the primal father Freud theorizes in *Totem and Taboo* (2012), the incest taboo, and the analogous neglect of the mother, are problems Lacan inherits and does not solve. The incest taboo of concern to Freud (and, also, to Lacan but in a different way) separates the boy from the m/Other. In Ettinger's summary, the Freudian myth "produces desire as repressed and infinitely displaced…Desire, and the subject, both phallic and patterned on the boy's repression of the maternal body, are supposed to account for desire and subject in general" (2006d, 96). Multiple questions are thus left unanswered. We do not know how to account for the girl's desire. Nor do we know, as Lacan acknowledges, how to account for the "prohibition of incest between father and daughter" (Lacan 2006c, 619). Ettinger adds, by way of critique, that the incest taboo and paternal function only, fully, operate for the boy, and yet the analytic of desire developed by Lacan is not specific to the boy, but generalized to everyone. The incest taboo is based on the experience of the Oedipal-boy and the girl-daughter's own unique experience of the incest prohibition in the phallic domain and, also, in the matrixial (pre-birth incest), is occluded. The problem dates back to Freud's analytic myth relating to the totemic Father. He is imagined from the vantage point of the boy-son-becoming man and not from the vantage point of the daughter-girl-becoming woman (or possible future mother).

In the Lacanian theorization, everyone suffers from symbolic castration. Both girls and boys must relinquish their attachments to "corporeality, to bodily organs quo partobject and to the archaic m/Others" (Ettinger 1997, 373). But because the boy's organ is symbolized he must give up what he appears to have in the imaginary. The girl, by contrast, must give up what she does not have because there is no symbolization of the girl-woman's sex. In Ettinger's summation, "Men confront the question of having/not-having the phallus, and women, on top of that, of being/not-being a phallic objet a of desire for men" (374). Lacan's analytic regards the desire and jouissance of the mother as largely threatening to the child and he fails, in Ettinger's estimate, to develop an account of what she calls pre-birth incest (which is not synonymous with after-birth incest that is, by definition, traumatic).

In the OSD, Ettinger finds an-Other desire, a Feminine desire based on what she calls the "non-prohibited incestuous in/outside rapport, interlaced between the becoming-subject and the archaic m/Other-to-be" (376). Pre-birth (or matrixial) incest is unavoidable and cannot be subject to paternal prohibition. The pre-birth incestuous encounter between the becoming-mother and the becoming-subject sets the Feminine-matrixial trans-subjective relation into play. The trans-subjective refers to "subjectivity-as-an-encounter" and, also, to an "enlarged subjectivity" in the matrixial. It must be remembered that Ettingerian theory gives Feminine pride of place to the subject-as-several (as distinct from the individual as One). She explains that the OSD is predicated upon "several/trans-subjectivity and hybrid objects, and informs an-Other desire" (368).

Unlike what Ettinger calls "genital-phallic Oedipal sexual incest" (2006d, 142) which is harmful and destructive, matrixial incest is life begetting and unavoidable. Matrixial incest is about a seduction into life. As such, it is erotic and generates a sexual relation in the borderlinking. Griselda Pollock (2013) helpfully explains that matrixial Eros involves "yearning to experience connectivity and besideness with an unknown yet intimate other" (183). Desire in the matrixial is about the "psychic capacity for differentiation-in-coemergence and separation-in-jointness, where distance-in-proximity is continuously reattuned" (Ettinger 2001, 127). A crucial difference between the Lacanian and Ettingerian formulation of desire as related to the Other/archaic-mother is with respect to the way the former is singular (referring to the desire of the Other) and the latter is plural (referring to webbed desire, the woman-m/Other as assemblage, and this desire as composite). Additionally, matrixial desire is not integrated into or offset by the Name of the Father (or paternal function) theorized by Lacan. Matrixial desire, as noted above, is non-Oedipal and un-cut by the signifier. It includes "traces of partially foreclosed feminine-maternal incest in search of ways to become known" (Ettinger 2006d, 107).

Although anyone, regardless of sexual morphology, can occupy the position of m/Other, the "prenatal maternal figure is always female, and the imprints of the contact with this female figure will infiltrate any maternal figure, be it the same or another person" (Ettinger 2006a, 70). The corpo-Reality of the birth-giving mother is significant in matrixial terms. "The first corporeal-psychic connection between *I* and *non-I* occurs inside the maternal womb where every I is in linkage with the female invisible corporeality and is borderlinking to the m/Other's psychic environment" (70). Ettinger is not, in my reading, trying to essentialize the birth-giving mother or intending to negate transgender identifications, including the experiences of transgender men who give birth, but naming something concerning the body that is, by definition, beyond words, pre-linguistic and better understood as Real. There is, in the non-conscious (and unsignifiable) experience of late-stage pregnancy and birth psychic and corpo-Real imprints that are shared and cross-inscribed. Differentiation and co-emergence in these originary moments recalls and is predicated upon the archaic Woman-m/Other as first *non-I* in a trans-subjective matrixial alliance.

This is what allows Ettinger to state that sexual difference in the matrixial is not about an opposition or difference between the One and the Other, the masculine (all) and the feminine (not-all) for example, but about severality. Matrixial sexual difference involves an aggregated subjectivity (which Ettinger also calls severality) whereby the partial-subject exists in relation to other partial-subjects in shared matrixial webs.

What is important to understand here is that for Ettinger pregnancy is not based on fusion, symbiosis or psychosis. Nor is it regressive. For Ettinger, the encounter-event of gestation enables trans-subjectivity (borderlinkings to Others as *non-I's*) and to sub-subjectivity (the Other(s) within me). While a sexual relationship is impossible in Lacanian terms, it co-occurs in the matrixial borderspace where we do not exist without Others (*non-I's*). In this transgressive matrixial space, the "I conjoins in the Real the jouissance of the body of *non-I*" (Ettinger 2006d, 142). As such, there is a Feminine sexual relation in the matrixial space of the non-phallic incestuous encounter event that inscribes sub-knowledge as matrixial imprints. The matrixial co-efficient is about inter-human connectivity, hybridity, co-affectivity, metramorphosis and attunement to the Other in the I (and the I in the Other): it is a non-regressive transitivity. In fact, transitivity is a sexual difference in the matrixial. Sex difference in the matrixial is not about the One (and its binary oppositions between object and subject), but about "thinking transmissivity and co-affectivity" (183). To put this in another way, the matrixial borderspace is a paradigm for thinking about the Feminine axis of difference in non-phallic and in non-psychotic terms.

What is most significant to Ettinger's theory of pre-birth incest is that it provides a basis for the OSD. This is, for Ettinger, the essence of Feminine sexual difference, the difference between the becoming-subject and the m/Other. Despite the fact that this axis of sexual difference is first and primary it has not been given substantive attention in psychoanalytic theory. As Ettinger explains, Feminine prenatal jouissance remains taboo or under theorized in the psychoanalytic corpus. Freud theorizes the incest taboo in relation to the law of the father but does not develop comparable theorizing in relation to the pregnant woman's body. "Her incest must occur in the Real, to give life, and therefore it cannot be forbidden on the one hand, and is supposed to signify nothing on the other hand" (Ettinger 1997, 387). There is, for Ettinger, a matrixial repression that emerges, in part, through intrauterine phantasies but also in "post-partum psychosis and infantile autism" (388) that is suggestive of "symbiotic fusion, splitting rejection, or persecutory rapport to the *non-I* [m/Other]" (388). Pre-birth incest is dangerous because it is unavoidable but also because it involves a realm of experience "beyond/before the separating line of castration, beyond/before the threshold of language" (388).

Conclusion

What Ettinger stresses in her formulation of the OSD is that we differ first and foremost from another woman-as-mother. Boys and girls alike, regardless of gender identity, trans- or cisgender status, must first negotiate a Feminine sexual difference from the m/Other before Oedipal sexual difference becomes a question and sexual positions relating to the desire of the Other and jouissance are established. The late pre-birth encounter-event with "female corporeal specificity produces for men and women a different, non-Oedipal sublimation where, in the search for *non-I's*, the *jouissance* is of the borderlinking itself" (Ettinger 2001, 110). There is always a relation between the one and the more than one Neill 2008 in the pre-birth incestuous liaison. This explains why the first sexual difference is with-in and between the *I* and the m/Other (as first *non-I*). As I will explain more thoroughly in the following chapters, there is a "shareable dimension of subjectivity" where both *I* and *non-I* "co-emerge and co-inhabit a joint space" (Ettinger 2006d, 65). But suffice here to say that the becoming-subject and the alterity of the mother exist in a non-unified sexual relation. This matrixial relation is not about feminine gender identity. Nor is it about sexual positioning in Lacanian terms, but a "pre-subjective difference" (Neill 2008, 330) that gives rise to the OSD.

In the following chapter on the Ettingerian Woman, I consider what Lacan does say about the m/Other, the womb, procreation, and the preverbal to more fully situate the matrixial-Feminine of relevance to the matrixial borderspace.

Bibliography

Anzieu, Didier, and Chris Trans Turner. 1989. The skin ego. Yale University Press.

Cavanagh, Sheila L. 2016. Transsexuality as Sinthome: Bracha L. Ettinger and the Other (Feminine) Sexual Difference. *Studies in Gender and Sexuality* (Abingdon) 17 (1): 27–44. https://doi.org/10.1080/15240657.2016.1135681.

Ettinger, Bracha Lichtenberg. 1992. Matrix and Metramorphosis. *Differences: A Journal of Feminist Cultural Studies* 4 (3): 176–209.

Ettinger, Bracha. 1997. The Feminine/Prenatal Weaving in Matrixial Subjectivity-as-Encounter. *Psychoanalytic Dialogues* 7 (3): 367–405.

Ettinger, Bracha. 2001. Matrixial Gaze and Screen: Other Than Phallic and Beyond the Late Lacan. In *Bodies of Resistance: New Phenomenologies of Politics, Agency, and Culture*, ed. Laura Doyle. Northwestern University Press.

Ettinger, Bracha. 2002. From Transference to the Aesthetic Paradigm: A Conversation with Félix Guattari. In *A Shock to Thought: Expression after Deleuze and Guattari*, ed. Brian Massumi. Routledge.

Ettinger, Bracha L. 2006a. Fascinance and the Girl-to-M/Other Matrixial Feminine Difference. In *Psychoanalysis and the Image*, ed. Griselda Pollock. Blackwell Publishing Ltd.

Ettinger, Bracha. 2006d. *The Matrixial Borderspace*, Theory out of Bounds. Vol. 28. University of Minnesota Press.

Ettinger, Bracha Lichtenberg. 2007. Diotima and the Matrixial Transference: Psychoanalytical Encounter-Event as Pregnancy in Beauty. In *Beyond the Threshold: Explorations of Liminality in Literature*, ed. Hein Viljoen and Chris N. Van der Merwe. Peter Lang.

Lacan, Jacques. 1992. *The Ethics of Psychoanalysis 1959–1960: The Seminar of Jacques Lacan*. Edited by Jacques-Alain Miller. Translated by Dennis Porter. Book VII. W. W. Norton & Company Inc.

Lacan, Jacques. 1997. *The Seminar of Jacques Lacan: The Psychoses 1955–1956, Book III*. Reprint edition. Translated by Jacques-Alain Miller and Russell Grigg. Norton.

Lacan, Jacques. 2006a. Remarks on Daniel Lagache's Presentation: "Psychoanalysis and Personality Structure. In *Écrits: The First Complete Edition in English*. Translated by Bruce Fink. W.W. Norton & Company.

Lacan, Jacques. 2006b. Response to Jean Hyppolite's Commentary on Freud's "Verneinung". In *Écrits: The First Complete Edition in English*. Translated by Bruce Fink. W.W. Norton & Company.

Lacan, Jacques. 2006c. Guiding Remarks for a Conversation on Female Sexuality. In *Écrits: The First Complete Edition in English*, translated by Bruce Fink. W.W. Norton & Company.

Lacan, Jacques. 2006d. Seminar on "The Purloined Letter". In *Écrits: The First Complete Edition in English*. Translated by Bruce Fink. W.W. Norton & Company.

Lacan, Jacques. 2020. *Jacques Lacan: The Object Relation*. The Seminar of Jacques lacan, Book IV. Edited by Jacques-Alain Miller. English Translation. Polity.

Morel, Geneviève. 2018. *The Law of the Mother: An Essay on the Sexual Sinthome*. 1st ed. Routledge.

Neill, Calum. 2008. Severality: Beyond the Compression of the Cogito. *Subjectivity* 24 (1): 325–339. https://doi.org/10.1057/sub.2008.21.

Pollock, Griselda. 2013. Art as Transport-Station of Trauma? Haunting Objects in the Works of Bracha Ettinger, Sarah Kofman and Chantal Akerman. In *Representing Auschwitz: At the Margins of Testimony*. Springer.

Schilder, Paul. 2013. *The Image and Appearance of the Human Body*. Routledge.

4

The Ettingerian Woman

Bracha L. Ettinger is critical of the way the Woman does not exist in Lacan's theory of sexuation. In his formulation, the "Woman" is not-all subject to the phallic premise while the man is all subject to the phallic premise. As a result, part of the Woman's being is in excess of the Symbolic. Contra Lacan, the Woman fully exists in Ettinger's theory of the matrixial borderspace. In this chapter, I outline Ettinger's critique of Lacan and Freud vis-à-vis Feminine sexuality, explicate her formulation of Woman from the vantage of the matrixial, and consider how her formulation of Woman sits alongside Lacan's writings on the Other and the inter-said. In so doing, I ask if the Ettingerian Woman is not the Lacanian Other inclusive of the intra-said [*intra-dit*]. My intention is not to collapse Ettingerian psychoanalysis into Lacanian theory, but to read Ettinger's writings on Woman alongside Lacan's teachings to parse out what is truly new in her theorization. Before I consider how Ettinger does say more about the Woman from the perspective of the matrixial, let us first consider her critique of both Freud and Lacan in more depth.

Ettinger gives sustained attention to Lacan's later writings on unconscious sexuality where he explores Feminine sexuality and the Woman who does not exist. Lacan freely admits in his seminar on Feminine

S. L. Cavanagh, *Bracha L. Ettinger and Jacques Lacan*, The Palgrave Lacan Series,
https://doi.org/10.1007/978-3-032-23293-9_4

sexuality that the "not-whole…[is] obviously giving me a hard time" (Lacan 1998, 57). In other words, the "not-whole" is where the Woman escapes Lacan's understanding. He aligns the Woman with truth and admits to not knowing. "I don't know how to approach, why not say it, the truth – no more than woman. I have said that the one and the other are the same thing, at least to man. They constitute the same conundrum (*embarrass*)" (120). Despite not-knowing, Lacan arrives at a conclusion: the Woman does not exist as One because she is not-all subject to the phallic premise (as signifier). In other words, something in her *ex-ists*. By this, Lacan means that she is beyond the Symbolic coordinates established by the signifying structure. This is what gives her access to an Other (non-phallic) jouissance in his sexuation theory. But more than this, the Lacanian Woman who does not exist is a symptom of man. She is also his object cause of desire, the *Thing* (*das Ding*) around which his search for knowledge pivots. Insisting that he relishes both, woman and truth, Lacan says that the "discordance between knowledge and being is my subject" (120). The lack of knowledge and understanding drives the "game of encore" (120), the search for a better jouissance. Ettinger does not offer Lacan a better jouissance, but she does offer a formulation of the Woman who does exist from the perspective of the matrixial. Let us consider her critical addendum to the Lacanian model of unconscious sexuality.

For Ettinger, there is a discourse and aesthetic particular to the Feminine that is submerged in Lacanian theorizing and in modernity more generally. More specifically, Ettinger is concerned about the status of the Woman and the Feminine in Lacanian theory. Her critical question is about how the Feminine figures as supplementary in Lacanian psychoanalysis when it is, in fact, primary. She is, ultimately, asking if the non-existent Woman is a structural fact of life that Lacan interprets, or if he repeats a problem, the very problem he seeks to solve, relating to the Woman who does not exist, in his own theorizing, For Ettinger, it is a bit of both. She contends that Feminine heterogeneity is not registered in the phallic axis in a way that would be "independent from the *all* to which it is related and from the experience to which it is *supplementary*" (Ettinger 2000c, 188). By this, she means to suggest that the Feminine axis of difference cannot be registered from the perspective of the "all" (the man's side), because it is not bound to the phallic signifier. But, to complicate matters, Lacan repeats the problem of what we might call the disappearing Woman in his theory of sexuality by failing to say more about the Feminine not-all.

Freud and Lacan

Lacan's contention that the Woman does not exist is, for Ettinger, not unlike Freud's inability to theorize the Feminine as anything but passive and masochistic. In Ettinger's critique of Freud, she notes that the girl's sexuality is, for Freud, essentially masculine: he refers to little girls as little boys in the pregenital stages. Moreover, the genital stage is named phallic because it is the penis that orchestrates sexual difference (Ettinger 1997, 372–373).

To his credit, Lacan is critical of the anatomical approach to sexual difference built into Freudian psychoanalysis. His solution is to interpret Freud's theory of sexuality linguistically, thereby viewing the phallus as a signifier as opposed to an organ. The phallus is, for Lacan, a faulty signifier or, rather, a signifier of lack. It is not the *Thing* it is meant to represent. Rather, the phallus demarcates an absence. Lacan develops his theory of sexuation on the basis of two distinct ways of being in relation to a fundamental lack. One can either be the phallus or have the phallus (in phantasy), assuming a Feminine or masculine position respectively. The position one chooses to inhabit in relation to the phallus as signifier is contingent, not biologically determined. There are, for Lacan, only two ways of living with lack (castration). One can choose a Feminine or masculine solution, not both. Either way, something relating to being does not get inscribed in the Symbolic. There is nothing to designate what Lacan calls the "bipolarity of sex." Activity and passivity as theorized by Freud—who wrote that libido is always active—does not resolve the question of unconscious sexual difference and Lacan understands this.

The two divergent relations to the phallic premise are, for Lacan, unreal (and beyond signification). But the man is fully inscribed in the Symbolic whereas the Woman is not-all inscribed in the Symbolic; something about her being falls out of signifying order. This is what Lacan explicates in his formula on sexuation: the man cultivates the fantasy that he has the phallus, whereas the woman cultivates the fantasy that she is the phallus: two divergent relations to what is, for Lacan, the inaugural signifier. The man is all inscribed while the woman is not-all inscribed by the phallic signifier. To the extent that the "man" has the phallus and the "woman" is the phallus, the metonymy linking the penis (as organ) to phallus (as signifier) remains in play. Ettinger's main critique is that Lacan repeats the Freudian problem of not being able to account for the girl-woman without recourse to the phallic signifier. She says: "Lacan's famous statement, that (the) woman does not exist and does not signify anything [because she is not fully subject to the phallic premise], echoes Freud's remark on the prepubertal nonexistence of femaleness, and on the pre-Oedipal maternal obscurity" (Ettinger 2006d, 96).

Ettinger contends that for Lacan, the "phallus is the only imaginary representation of sex-difference…and castration is the only passageway to significance" (1997, 372). While Lacan is clear about the fact that sexual difference cannot be represented (and that he is trying to represent what lacks signification), he does adopt the phallus which is metonymically related to the penis (as organ) to establish sexual difference in his model. Like Freud before him who regarded the presence or absence of the penis as the thing upon which sexual difference hinges, Lacan understands the Feminine within the phallic orbit. It follows that the Woman is, for Lacan, a "hole in the Real and the Symbolic" (Ettinger 2006d, 73). In Lacanian theory, the Woman does not exist because she is in-excess of the phallic premise. In Ettinger's assessment of Lacanian theory, it is limited to the extent that he cannot articulate a sexual difference beyond the phallic register. Her major point of contention is that psychoanalytic theory has not yet succeeded in articulating a Feminine axis of difference beyond the phallic premise; an axis of matrixial difference that can apprehend the Woman.

Although Lacan, like Freud, gives us many important psychoanalytic tools to theorize desire, sexuality, the Other, and jouissance, they repeatedly fail, in Ettinger's estimate, to ascertain a space for the girl-becoming-Woman that is not already passive (as Freud tells us) or non-existent (as Lacan tells us). For Ettinger, the truth of the "Woman" is only half-told in Lacan's oeuvre because his writing is delimited by the phallus—even as it is, for Lacan, a signifier of imprecise meaning and not a piece of flesh. Ettinger explains that Lacan defines the Woman as Other (to man), as *Thing* and as symptom (of man). In her view, women are objects of exchange in the Lacanian frame (Ettinger 1997, 367). The Woman is the non-object cause of man's desire which appears to be there but is not. As such, the Woman is man's (fantasy) symptom (or sinthomatic support). Ettinger is troubled by the way the Woman is reduced to "Woman-Other-Thing" in Lacan's discourse. She is "constituted as a fetish, like an inanimate object, first absent and desired and later inspired, by some imagined breath, to come to life, like a Golem, now present and possessed" (Ettinger 2006d, 176).

Let us be clear about the fact that while Ettinger critiques Lacan for his phallocentrism she does not contest the existence of the phallic order he theorizes. She contends that his interpretation of it is elaborated from the man's side. She is critical of the way the Woman is reduced to an object (as in *object a*), to a symptom, and to a radical otherness beyond apprehension in his teachings. She elaborates:

> Whether a Woman-Other-thing, a product of the Real's non-sense, whether a radical Other, whether dangerously bordering on originary repression of the Thing, whether equated with an elusive almost-nothing (*objet a*) – even when described as 'not all,' the concept of woman as defined in the Lacanian psychoanalysis is always automatically reinforcing the Phallic structure because 'woman' is perceived as the holes in this structure, its scraps, rests, excess or surplus. (2000c, 187)

By this, she means that while the Woman is not inscribed in the Symbolic she, nevertheless, lends support to it. In Ettinger's formulation, Woman's lack in the "Real inscribes a lack in the Symbolic" (1997, 373) that must be understood from the perspective of the matrixial. The lack in the (phallic) Symbolic leaves a trace connection to the matrixial. In other words, the Woman is an absent presence in a Symbolic chain—even as she is, paradoxically, beyond meaning. Difference functions as an absence and as Feminine in Lacan's formulation. But for Ettinger, the Feminine "enters subjectivity as the alterity of *transitivity and jointness* – not of *absolute Other*" (2006b, 112).

Masculine sexuality, as distinct from Feminine sexuality, is, for Lacan, about *object a* (as non-object cause of desire). The man does not look for an actual woman but for the *a*, "the true object, for what's at stake in desire, which isn't the Other, but this leftover" (Lacan 2014, 198). In other words, masculine desire for the Other-woman has little, if anything, to do with actual women. It is delimited by a fundamental fantasy about the way the m/Other (as first Other) lacks or seems, retroactively, to have been lost. Feminine sexuality is about an Other jouissance that is Real (unsymbolizable). As Bruce Fink suggests, the Other jouissance responds to "a lack in the Other as real" (Fink 2002). Let us consider the lack in the Other as real in relation to the Lacanian Woman.

The Lacanian Woman Does Not Exist

Lacan caused great controversy in Paris and in international psychoanalytic circles when he said that the Woman does not exist. Lacan writes that "*woman* does not exist, woman is *not whole* (*pas toute*) – woman's sexual organ is of no interest (*ne lui dit rien*) except via the body's jouissance…woman is defined by a position that I have indicated as "not whole" (*pas-tout*) with respect to phallic jouissance" (1998, 7). Understandably, his comments on the Woman who does not exist provoked great feminist uproar, discussion and debate in and out of psychoanalysis. Some Lacanian-inspired feminist psychoanalytic theorists view Lacan's theory of the non-existent Woman as a structural fact due, in part, to the way we are cut by language and alienated by the signifier (Barnard 2002; Brousse 2022; Copjec 2004, 2015; Morel 2002, 2018; Ragland-Sullivan 2012; Soler 2006). Other feminists, by contrast, are troubled by what appears to be a structuralist approach whereby Lacan seems to lend analytic support to an essentialist or linguistically determined bi-gender heteronormative body politic (Butler 1992, 2011; Grosz 2002, 2017, 2020a, 2020b).[1]

We may not be able to resolve the question about whether Lacan is interpreting the structural facts of life relating to unconscious sexuality

[1] See Shanna De la Torre (2018) for a discussion of structuralism in Lacanian psychoanalysis.

linguistically or, alternatively, if he is colluding in a phallocentric logic that negates the Feminine. But it is productive to consider how Ettinger navigates the theoretical quagmire. Before I discuss Ettinger's critical feminist supplement to the Lacanian theory of sexuality, let us consider how he understands the Woman who does not exist in more specific detail. When Lacan writes that we cannot talk about "Woman" because she lacks a signifier, he is, in my view, not intending to be sexist so much as he is trying to convey that she is not-whole and thus in excess of the Symbolic. Due to this excess she experiences a supplementary jouissance which is not of the order of words, discourse or the signifier. This is how we must interpret Lacan's statement that the Woman has no universal value. He does not mean that women lack cultural value as subjects but, rather, that the Woman is in excess of the phallic premise and thus resists definitive inscription. There is something about the way the Women do not exist in full that is of Real significance to women. But suffice here to say that something about her being as other is in excess of the signifier and thus language.

This excess gives women access to an Other (non-phallic) jouissance, which, as Joan Copjec (2004) explains, "unglues her from her own body" (103). Unlike the man, a woman can experience an Other (Feminine) jouissance in addition to phallic (paltry) jouissance. It should also be noted that Lacan understands women to have a specific relation to the Other and that the un-glueing referred to by Copjec is due, in part, to her proximity to the Other. Lacan explains that "woman is that which has a relationship to that Other" (Lacan 1998, 81). Moreover, he contends that there is something about being the Other that is the province of the Woman alone in the unconscious. "Woman has a relation to the signifier of that Other, insofar as, qua Other, it can but remain forever Other" (Lacan 1998, 81). This is why women experience what Lacan calls an Other (Feminine) jouissance.

While everyone, regardless of sexual positioning, experiences (Real) bodily jouissance, women (as sexuated subjects) have a more complicated relation to bodily jouissance. This is due to the way elements of a woman's being lack inscription in the Symbolic. The man (as a sexuated subject), by contrast, can more easily sustain an illusion of wholeness. Consequently, women's position in the Symbolic is more tenuous. In

Lacanian terms, women are "not whole" or "not-all" subject to the phallic signifying apparatus, a linguistic system upon which what Lacan calls the Symbolic is based, whereas men are fully subject to it. Lacan writes that if she is:

> excluded by the nature of things, it is precisely that in being not all (not-whole), she has, in relation to what the phallic function designated of jouissance, a supplementray jouissance…It is not because she is not-all in the phallic function that she is not there at all. In relation to the phallic function she is *not* not there at all. She participates fully. But there is something more *[en plus]*.…she has her own *jouissance* of which she perhaps knows nothing, except that she experiences it – that, she knows. (Lacan 1975, 68–69, Quoted in Ettinger 2006d)

This Other jouissance is "symbolized by the body" (Lacan Lacan, 39) for Lacan but it also takes on a reality vis-à-vis the Real. This jouissance is in excess of language. It has nothing to do with "men" (87) and everything to do with the infinite (103).

Lacan explains that "It's not because she is not-wholley in the phallic function that she is not there at all. She is *not* not at all there. She is there in full (*à plein*). But there is something more (*en plus*)" (74). This "*en plus*" is jouissant. To put this in yet another way, the Woman is not wholly subject to the phallic function and women enjoy-suffer proportionately. When Lacan says that the Woman does not exist or that she is not One, he means that there is something in the Feminine experience that escapes the phallic signifier (72). This gives women something extra or, in Lacanian terms, "a leg up."

The man, by contrast, is fully subject to the phallic premise. His sexuality is not about the Other. Masculine "jouissance, qua sexual is phallic – in other words, it is not related to the Other as such" (9). The man will always miss the Woman (although she can be his symptom) because he desires something intangible, the object cause of his own desire (*object a*). Lacan explains that the man "never deals with anything by way of a partner but *object a*" (80). In his essay titled "Position of the Unconscious," Lacan explains the problem more precisely. He writes that "there is no access to the opposite sex as Other except via the so-called partial drives wherein the subject seeks an object to take the place of the loss of life he has sustained due to the fact that he is sexed" (2006f, 720).

It follows that there is no sexual relationship between men and women. Specifically, Lacan claims that "there's no such thing as a sexual relationship to be announced *as truth*" (1998, 12). He also says that the sexual relation fails because there is an imagined equivalence between the sexes from the man's side. This is to say that the man (One) does not relate to the woman. The Woman (as Other) is One-less (*l'Un-en-moins*). For Lacan, phallic enjoyment prohibits a "man" from enjoying a "woman's" body because his jouissance is of the organ, not of women per se. The jouissance had by men will never "conjoin organically" (2014, 265). In effect, it has little, if anything, to do with his woman-partner. Lacan does not say that men and women do not have sex or that there are not attempts at what we might call sexual relating from the man's side, but that from the perspective of masculine jouissance there is a structural inability to connect to the Woman.

The Ettingerian Woman

Ettinger responds to the curious position of the Woman in Lacan's teachings whereby she is related and unrelated to the phallic function. She is deeply critical of how the Woman is confined to a phallic stratum in Lacan's teachings and the way this model can only ascertain an "axis of the One and the Infinite, with its *same* and *oppositions*, all and nothing, as its surplus, residue, Other, impossibility, contingency" (Ettinger 2006d, 113). This contingency is due, in part, to the fact that there is, in Lacan's assessment, no "symbolization of woman's sex as such" (Lacan 1993, 176). She is forced to "take on the image of the other sex as the basis of its [her] identification" (176). In other words, her access to the Symbolic is less direct than it is for the "man" whose organ is symbolized. Woman is "characterized by an absence, a void, a hole" (176) which is not, according to Lacan, a "pure quirk of nature" (176).

As already noted, Ettinger is critical of the Lacanian reduction of Woman to a void, a *Thing*, a hole, or lack in the Real. Her theory of the matrixial is offered as a feminist supplement to what she calls the phallocentrism of Lacanian psychoanalysis. But let us be clear about the fact that Ettinger does not contest Lacan's theory of unconscious sexuality including the way the Woman does not exist from the man's side, or the way the woman's sex does not symbolize as such. Her theoretical contribution is a feminist *supplement* to the Lacanian formalization of sexual difference. Ettinger contends that there is another matrixial side from which the Woman does exist and her sex can be apprehended, if not symbolized directly. For Ettinger, the Woman must be something more than a man's symptom and does exist, albeit in an expanded sub-Symbolic where something beyond the word-image may appear. This appearance requires a matrixial gaze as distinct from a phallic gaze (to be discussed below), but Woman can, nevertheless, be discerned.

Through Ettinger's work we are able to see that it is not the Woman but rather the (phallic) Symbolic that is lacking. It cannot signify the Real. There is a gap between the Real and that which is registered by the Symbolic (language, cultural signs, symbols, etc.). The Symbolic should not be limited to whole and discrete signs, symbols and signifiers in Ettinger's view. There is, in other words, a matrixial sub-Symbolic that is eclipsed in Lacan's model of the (phallic) Symbolic. By attending to the sub-Symbolic, Ettinger develops a theory of the matrixial subject that escapes the Lacanian formulation (as discussed in the previous chapter). Her position is, to some extent, consistent with the French psychotherapist and semiologist, Félix Guattari, who notes, the "linguistic signifier in no way encloses all of the components combining to produce subjectivity" (quoted in Ettinger 2002, 244). Ettinger contends that we must find ways to understand subjectivity in an expanded Symbolic, one that can apprehend the Feminine. There must be a way to trace a Feminine prediscursive dimension that is before and beyond the signifier.

Before explicating Woman in the matrixial, let us be clear about what she is not. For Ettinger, Woman is not reducible to the mother, to the womb (as organ), or to natal female sex specificity. Nor is Woman an individual, an identity, or a radical alterity (Ettinger 2001, 129). Woman does not exist in the confines of any-one body. She is, for Ettinger, the site of an encounter-event in the matrixial borderlinking that is, from a Lacanian perspective, closely related to the Real of the body. What is especially difficult to grasp from a non-psychoanalytic gender studies perspective is the way the Ettingerian Woman is not intended to be a gendered construct (although it cannot help but be read as such because sex and gender categories dominate our linguistic lexicon). The Ettingerian Woman is developed as an alternative to sexual positioning in the Lacan frame which, while also not about gender identity, pertains to the register of the Imaginary and the Real. Ettinger's Woman designates different conditions of partial-subjective co-emergence that predate and operate alongside sexual positioning in the phallic domain theorized by Lacan. In order to avoid the reduction of Woman to an individual subject or, indeed to a gender identity, it may be helpful to remember that for Ettinger a father and son relation can be a Woman.

Importantly, Woman is also not a *Thing* (*das Ding*), as she is for Lacan, but an "other-Thing that lies beyond" (Ettinger 2006d, 175). Nor is she an object or symptom of man. For Ettinger, Woman is a Real non-linguistic predicate for borderlinkings in the matrixial. In other words, the Ettingerian Woman is a Real basis for all other psychical and phenomenological trace-like connections to others. The Woman exists in conditions of co-emergence between partial-subjects (Others and *non-I*'s) in asymmetrical non-conscious relations; these are encounter-events in the matrixial borderlinking that cannot be signified in the Symbolic as such. As Ettinger explains, Woman exists in the "field of Event and Encounter and as an almost-other-Event-Encounter that is borderlinked to the I" (Ettinger 2006d, 175). Thus, she cannot be an absolute Other. We are bound to others in difference and through matrixial cross-inscriptions which may be compared, in my view, to Lacan's explication of the signifying trace. Ettinger's Woman is a border-Other, a "*becoming in-ter-with the Other*, an *im-pure becoming-between in jointness*" (Ettinger 2006d, 112).

Ettinger's main psychoanalytic point is that Woman is a condition of transitivity, one that can be felt and apprehended. There is no one isolated subject in a matrixial web, only Woman, defined as a condition of co-emergent relations between partial-subjects. Ettinger's definition of partial-subjectivity, or the subject-as-several (severality), is not synonymous with the Lacanian notion of the subject. For Lacan, the subject is alienated by the signifier and defined by a degree of autonomy from the m/Other insofar as we are speaking subjects. The Other Sexual Difference

(OSD) related to the matrixial (discussed in the previous chapter), predates castration and sexuation. We are not, as Ettinger notes, "cut from lack," we "appear by disappearing" (Ettinger 2006d, 147). In her discussion of the matrixial gaze, Ettinger explains how we appear and disappear, fade-in and out as we assume new and unforeseen shapes and apparitions circumventing the phallic gaze and the cultural screen as theorized by Lacan.

The phallic gaze obliterates something of relevance to the matrixial that Ettinger elaborates upon in her discussion of Eurydice, a character in Greek mythology who was lost to life when caught by the gaze of Orpheus, her husband, who could not trust in her existence without laying his eyes upon her. The matrixial gaze (discussed in Chap. 1), by contrast, can intercept something of importance to one's history and destiny. The matrixial gaze re-installs the Feminine *as* a borderlinking. What Ettinger is getting at in her discussion of the matrixial gaze and in her formulation of Woman, is that there is something(s) relevant to our being that cannot be signified (seen or said), yet nevertheless exists. Part of what needs to be apprehended through what Ettinger calls compassionate atunnement is the way we are borderlinked to Others in our respective matrixial webs. Trace vibrations between partial-subjects can be felt and intuited, even as they are out of time and step with the (phallic) present. Ettinger imagines Woman to be a non-conscious borderlinking in the matrixial where we co-relate in asymmetrical and phantasmatic time-space encounters.

In the matrixial substratum Woman "digs an-other area of difference with its specific apparatus, processes, and functions" (Ettinger 1997, 367). This difference is felt-sensed-intuited through transmissions of affect, psychic traces, and through what Ettinger calls erotic aerials. Ettinger defines the trace as a somatic register or affective deposit made by/with an Other. We might understand Ettinger's affective trace inscriptions of jouissance in terms of Lacan's markers, or what he calls invasive signifiers, imprinted on the subject's body by the Other. The erotic aerial, or a-link, is a matrixial reconfiguration of Lacan's *object a*. It is a "trace of a borderlinking" (Ettinger 2006d, 56), a non-object of significance to the subject-as-several.

Griselda Pollock (2007) likens the erotic aerial to "unsighted eyes" (192), much like the blind prophet Tiresias in the Oedipal trilogy

(Cavanagh 2016, 2018, 2022) who can see-apprehend what those, like Oedipus, cannot see with eyes. The erotic antennae registers "imprints that return from others as traces and transmit a centerless matrixial gaze as a sieve-like veil or tissue" (Ettinger 2006d, 149). The phantasmic waves and affects transmitted and received are "echoes of archaic partial relations and of feminine *jouissance from before-as-beside* the phallic era" (Ettinger 2006d, 100).

What Tiresias can see from a matrixial angle is that something happened in the ancestral legacy of Oedipus that co-affects everyone in his family along with the city of Thebes. The unknown incestuous and patricidal transgression haunts Oedipus. I stress this here because it must be remembered that the Feminine dimension of concern to Ettinger is not a feminist utopia. It is laced by phantasy, history, and trauma. As Ettinger explains, "The potential is there [in the matrixial borderspace] for traumatic and destructive as well as ethical or aesthetic deposits of jouissance" (2006d, 18).[2] (In the final chapter, I use Ettinger's work on the Feminine-matrixial to illustrate what counts not only as (phallic) Oedipal tragedy, but a matrixial tragedy in the life story of Antigone (sister/daughter to Oedipus).) Ettinger's main point is that there is trauma and tragedy in the Feminine dimension worthy of psychoanalytic attention. In this book, I consider these traumata in the case of Dora, Lol Stein, and Antigone in Chaps. 5, 6 and 7, respectively. Suffice here to say here that the Feminine sexual relation involves an attunement to the traumas and legacies of the m/Other and to multiple others genetically related and not to the *I* whom cannot be forgotten.

The Others who cannot be forgotten are central to the Ettingerian definition of Woman. We do not exist as separate entities, or as individuals, in the Feminine dimension. Woman cannot be delimited by inner and outer polarities (Ettinger 2002, 236) as in, for example, inside and outside the individual-subject-body. In the Feminine axis of difference "Woman" emerges—not as a unitary figure, but as an intricate weave trans-connecting two (or more) others (as partial-subjects). Ettinger likens Woman to a plait and to a complex weave. She frequently uses textile

[2] It should be remembered that Ettinger's oeuvre is shaped by her familial experience of the German-Jewish Holocaust and the intergenerational-familial transmission of trauma.

metaphors to illustrate how the Woman is like an assemblage. Notably, Lacan also uses textile metaphors including, but not limited to, knots, buttonholes, and to quilting points to explain how the signifier functions like a "spatializing device" (Lacan 1993, 267). In *Seminar III*, Lacan likens the function of the father, for instance, to a "quilting point between the signifier and the signified" (268). The quilting point is, in other words, a point of insertion whereby the signifier and the signified are not coupled but knotted. In Lacan's early work on psychosis, he contends that these quilting points hold the subject together.

In Ettingerian theory, Woman is not (exactly) the quilting points of concern to Lacan, but a condition of co-emergence that is in excess of the quilt-like signifier. Her theorization incorporates the corporeality of the body more fully or, at least, differently. The corpo-Real in the matrixial is not reducible to the physical body because it involves phantasy and matrixial desire. It is linked to the Lacanian register of the Real but, in Ettinger's reformulation, not without sense. The corpo-Real, as elaborated by Ettinger, calls to mind a Deleuzian assemblage that mutates and changes form but not in a haphazard way. The assemblage takes shape alongside and in keeping with co-emergent relations with Others as heterogeneous partners in difference. Others and *non-I*'s are central to the corpo-Real in the matrixial. The corpo-Real exceeds the bounds of the Symbolic. But more importantly for Ettinger's project, female corpo-Reality does not signify in a unique way. This is to say that female sex difference inclusive of reproductive capacity is doubly absent. For Ettinger, the "female invisible bodily specificity [is] an issue of sex-difference in its own right for women" (Ettinger 1997, 374). She explains that "female bodily specificity is the…site, physically, imaginatively, and symbolically, where a feminine difference emerges, and through which a "woman" is interlaced as a figure that is not confined to one-body, but is rather a hybrid "webbing" of links between several subjectivities, who by virtue of that webbing become partial" (Ettinger 2006d, 141).

In Griselda Pollock's summation, "Woman means different conditions: not just object or subject but the structure of transitivity" (2004, 46). For Ettinger, Woman is a transitive sex difference. While transitivity is usually regarded as infantile and regressive in psychoanalysis because the difference between the subject and the other is assumed to be confused, for Ettinger transitivity is a sexual difference that is primary and not pathological (or psychotic). This Feminine transitivity is also not about symbiosis or fusion: It enables the *I* to maintain its integrity within a relation to the *non-I*. Sexual difference in the matrixial is a Feminine, originary, and primordial difference (Ettinger 1997, 370). It is also a condition of transitivism where what happens to me and what happens to you are inseparable. This is, in part, what Ettinger means when she talks about the subject-as-several (or severality): the subject bound to the Others joy and pain in difference.

As discussed in the previous chapter, the OSD is enabled by Woman which Ettinger also defines as the "*co-emerging partial self and the Other*, or a different kind of relations to the Other" (Ettinger 2006d, 72). As such, Woman in Ettingerian theory is neither an individual-subject or an object cause of desire for the man (as she is in Lacan). The Woman does not exist in the confines of any-one subject body. She is an "*Otherity: a partial alterity that infiltrates the I*" (2006d, 190). Another way to think about Woman is to imagine her as a border-creature or, rather, a "*border-Other*, a *becoming in-ter-with the Other*, an *im-pure becoming-between in jointness*" (2001, 72). This border-Other is a non-conscious support for the Feminine dimension. The matrixial-Feminine dimension is predicated upon un-cognized memories of the mother-to-be/subject-to-be encounter felt by those who will later become men and women. In the Feminine, subjects exist in relation to others (*non-I*'s). We change, become, and co-fade in distance and proximity to others in a common matrixial assemblage. "Assemblages composed of unknown *I*(s) and *non-I*(s), [are]...points of support for matrixial desire and knowledge" (Ettinger 2000b, 63).

By unearthing knowledge in the Real beyond the signifier, Ettinger gives us a paradigm for thinking about the late prenatal period as a matrixial borderspace of linking whereby the subject-to-be and the mother-to-be are relating and not fused. It is important to the Ettingerian project to theorize gestation and, by extension, the borderlinking as non-psychotic because she intends to posit an account of the subject-as-several without recourse to non-sense. Severality is about the way we are bound to Others in difference. Another way to make the point is to say that what counts as Woman in Ettinger's theorization is that part of all of us that is uniquely attuned to the trauma in the Other (as Real) in the borderlinking. In Ettinger's oeuvre, the subject is not only alienated and internally split (as they are in the Lacanian Symbolic), but trans-subjectively tethered to multiple Others (*non-I's*) in the matrixial sub-Symbolic. The Woman is, for Ettinger, the anchoring point not only for the OSD, but is used to illustrate the way we are trans-connected to Others, known and unknown, in shared matrixial webs.

As indicated above, the Lacanian focus on the phallic signifier repeats the problem of the Oedipal-castration model that absents the Woman and the m/Other in Ettinger's critique. As she explains, the Lacanian phallus

> mainly stands for a symbolic principle: it is the signifier of signifiers *and* of difference—or of difference conceived *as* absence. But it is also the only imaginary representation of sex difference, and "castration" is the only passageway to symbolic significance, where oppositions and exclusions resonate. (Ettinger 2006d, 96)

It follows, in Ettinger's critique, that the Other is alienated in the Lacanian focus on the signifier. Not only does this preclude a sexual rapport on what Ettinger calls the Feminine side, but it does not make theoretical sense. How can the Other's desire in the subject function without a corresponding theory of intrasubjectivity in the Real? In other words, Ettinger asks how are we to understand what the desire and phantasy of the Other means in Lacan when he does not offer a formulation of intrasubjectivity whereby the desire of the Other could meet the trauma and jouissance of the I.

> In the classical Lacanian theory, it is not the phantasy of the subject that reflects the phantasy of the Other, but rather the desire of the subject that reflects the desire of the Other. Trauma is individual, and phantasy is in correlation with a *jouissance assumed to be* in the realm of the Other. In what sense may one formulate the desire of the Other in direct and positive relation to the *jouissance* of the subject, if desire is a concept that "kills" *jouissance*, and if the Other is an alienated network of chains of signifiers? (Ettinger 2006d, 103–104)

Ettinger's question about how the desire of the Other comes to resonate for the subject in Lacanian theory is important. For Ettinger and others interested in the transmission of desire, phantasy, and jouissance, there is an outstanding question in Lacanian psychoanalysis about how to understand the interrelation between the Other and the subject when there is, as Lacan is fond of saying, no sexual relation.

Is There a Sexual Relation with the Other?

Ettinger delves deep into Lacanian psychoanalysis to answer the question about how to understand the Other in the subject without recourse to sexual relating. Specifically, she focuses on Lacan's writings on the Woman and the Other in his later works. Ettinger's definition of Woman involving the "I with/for *some* other(s)" (Ettinger 2006d, 116) is developed in close relation to Lacan's formulation of the Other-imposed. Of this Other-imposed, Ettinger writes:

> The *between* involved in sexual rapport but displaced and…[the] *Other imposed*. To *Other-impose*, and it is curious that in imposing this Other, what I advanced today concerns *only* the woman. And it is she who, in this figure of the Other, gives us an illustration…to be, as a poet has written, "between center and absence," between the meaning she take from what I've called the *at-least-one*, between the center as pure existence or *jouis-presence* and absence…which I could not write but to define as "Not-all" that which is not included in the phallic function, yet which is not its negation…absence which is no less *jouissance* than being *jouis-absence*. (Lacan 1972 quoted in Ettinger 1997, 389)

Ettinger's reading and reformulation of the Lacanian Other-imposed gives us a way to understand not only the way the Other is, in Lacan's terms, implicated in, for example, the intra-said, but also how to understand the "center" and "absence" differentiating the woman from the man. This is to say that the matrixial enables us to understand the "absence" (or "nothing" as Ettinger says) as the "focus of prohibition on the elusive feminine/prenatal incestual rapport, a lack based on its castrating foreclosure in the phallic paradigm" (389–390).

From the vantage point of the matrixial, the sexual rapport does not occur between two bodies (a man and the Woman, for instance), but between the I and some Others (*non-I*'s) in the borderlinking. The OSD in the matrixial apprehends "differences in the linking in-between *I* and *non-I* – not a difference (same or opposite) *from* the *non-I*" (2004, 89). In the matrix Woman is a "border-Other, a becoming in-ter-with the Other, never a radical alterity" (2001, 129). Ettinger's formulation of "an-other Other" (Ettinger 2006d, 104) is not circumscribed by the signifier, discourse, and the Symbolic. She further notes that Woman is "*not the Other* but the *co-emerging partial self and Other*, or a different kind of *relations* to the Other" (Ettinger 2006d, 72). We may interpret the co-emergence as a non-conscious co-occurrence in a phenomenological field that has Real psychic significance. The Other in me and the I in the Other cross-pollinate in ways that are not only subjectifying, but essential to life and to being in the Feminine dimension.

Ettinger is concerned with how the phantasy and desire of the Other reaches the subject if there is, as we see in Lacan, no linkage between the "subject's trauma and phantasy (axis of the Real) to the Other's desire (axis of the Symbolic)" (Ettinger 2006d, 104). Ettinger's solution is to posit a non-phallic Feminine relation whereby partial subjects (*I*'s and *non-I*'s) correspond in an asymmetrical field of difference she names the matrixial borderspace. In the matrixial borderspace Ettinger refers to a "matrixial convenant of severality" (Ettinger 2006d, 104) whereby other-Others (or partial subjects, *non-I*'s) co-relate and trans-connect. Trans-connectivity does not refer to transgender identity but to a "matrixial field of severality" (Ettinger 2006d, 108).[3] This field of severality enables Ettinger to posit an archaic-m/Other (at the level of phantasy) who is an other-Other. This other-Other is a *non-I* who is beyond and also "inter-with-in" (Ettinger 2006d, 106) the subject. The desire, trauma, and jouissance of the m/Other is transported to the becoming-subject through the matrixial portal.

[3] For a discussion of the relationship between the Ettingerian trans-subjective and transgender studies See: Cavanagh (2022).

Given the porousness of the matrixial web as it pertains to partial-subjects, transitivity is about subjectivity as encounter (not regression). Indeed, transitivity *is* a sexual difference in the matrixial. It should be noted that in his discussion of subjectivity and the "inter-said," Lacan posits a place "between-two-subjects" (Lacan 2006g, 677) which is, in my view, the original formulation of what Ettinger will later calls severality or the subject-as-encounter. What Ettinger calls matrixial subjectivity is founded upon a desire to respect the Other in the other but also the Other in the self-subject (sub-subjectivity). But desire does not depend upon loss and lack in the matrixial and differs from the Lacanian formulation of desire's non-object as subjectively unattainable. It should also be stressed that Ettinger's theory of matrixial subjectivity is not about inter-subjectivity whereby subjects consciously and intentionally interact. Intersubjectivity involves our relations with significant others (actual mothers and fathers, for example), while matrixial subjectivity involves partial-subjects, *non-I*'s, and others in a non-conscious zone or matrixial sub-stratum. This form of subjectivity involves a being in and with the Other, a non-conscious positioning with the internally divided subject (Ettinger 2006d, 151). It occurs on the subconscious Feminine plain.

This subconscious Feminine plain is where (and when) a sexual rapport may occur. While Ettinger faults Lacan for refusing to relent upon his claim that there is no sexual relationship, he does, in fairness, question his own position. Consider that Lacan writes, in his Seminar on Feminine sexuality, that "If there is some angle from which this business of the sexual relationship could be clarified, it's precisely from the ladies' side (côté), insofar as it is on the basis of the elaboration of the not-whole that one must break new ground" (Lacan 1998, 57). Lacan's apparent certainty about the sexual impasse is shadowed by interesting equivocations and qualifiers. He also says that while the "whole world talks about it [the sexual relationship not working out]" (32), it does find its own way to come about. What is most significant from an Ettingerian perspective is the way he comes to think about the sexual rapport in familial and generational terms. In 1978, a few years before his death, Lacan adds a relational and temporal twist to the sexual aporia. He writes in an unpublished manuscript titled "*Le moment de conclure*" (Quoted in Lacan Book XXV, 1977–1978[4]):

> I stated by putting it in the present tense that there is no sexual rapport. That is the basis of Psychoanalysis…There is no sexual rapport except for neighbouring generations; namely, parents on the one hand, and children on the other. That's what the interdiction of incest wards off (Quoted in Ettinger 1997, 389).[5]

What Lacan begins to articulate in what has been termed the "Final Lacan" (as distinct from the "Late Lacan")[6] is the way the sexual rapport does not exist in the time of the present. This suggests that there may be, outside the time of the present, a sexual rapport between what Ettinger calls partial-subjects (the *I* with their *non-I's*). Equally significant is the fact that Lacan locates the sexual impasse between men and women in the present. The sexual aporia is about the "impossibility of inscribing the sexual relationship between two bodies of different sexes" (Lacan 1998, 120) in the present tense.

This out-of-time sexual rapport is formalized in Ettinger's writing on matrixial time. The matrixial sexual relation occurs in another-time. Ettinger writes that the "desire to join-in-difference and differentiate-in-co-emergence with the Other…[involves] a joining with-in the other's trauma that echoes back to my archaic traumas" (Ettinger 2006d, 147). Recall also that the matrixial borderspace is an amalgam of trans-sensorial affects, aesthetics, and intuitions from different times: times that have been and times that have never been. The time and space of the matrixial links us to Others (*non-I's*), to generations past (inclusive of subjects we have never met), and to something beyond us (as individuals) (Ettinger 1994). As Lone Bertelsen (2004) explains in his reading of Ettinger, her

[4] See: Lacan, Jacques. 1977. 'Seminar XXV The Moment to Conclude (1977–1978): From 15th November 1977: Jacques Lacan'. Translated by Cormac Gallagher. With Julia Evans. LacanianWorks, November 15. https://lacanianworks.org/seminar-xxv-the-moment-to-conclude-1977-1978-begins-15th-november-1977-jacques-lacan.

[5] Ettinger references an unpublished manuscript titled "*Le moment de conclure.*"

[6] See Johnston, Adrian. "Lacan's endgame: Philosophy, science, and religion in the final seminars." *Crisis and Critique* 6.1 (2019): 157–187.

formulation of the matrixial involves a "discordance of different times" (141).

There is also, in Ettinger's formulation of time, a corpo-Real difference between girls and boys. Females have access to what Ettinger calls the "in-side and future-site" of the womb whereas both the girls and boys have access to an "out-site/past-side" (Ettinger 2006d, 143). The "in-side and future-site" is based on the Real and imagined potentiality of pregnancy, for the girl. The "out-side/past-side" is open to boys and girls because everyone, from a matrixial angle, has access to a borderlinking with the m/Other. From the perspective of the matrixial, females have more direct access to a "paradoxical time where the future traumatically meets the past, and to this paradoxical site where outside meets inside" (Ettinger 2006d, 182). Males, by semi-contrast, remain outside, "totally-outside and too-early…forever too late to access" (Ettinger 2006d, 143) the archaic space and time of potentiality. The position of the girl-woman and potential future mother to the in-side and future-site of the womb is not structurally advantageous. Much like the Other jouissance in the Lacanian paradigm gives women access to an other form of enjoyment, this enjoyment is also about suffering and not something that can be quantified as a sociological benefit. I would also note here that the traumatic moment where the future meets the past (referred to above) is not about a melancholic retention of time as, for example, Felix Guattari imagines it. Rather, Ettinger is referring to a matrixial formulation of "time-slowing with-in space" (Ettinger 2019, 29).

This time-slowing with-in space is core to Ettinger's imagining of the *I* and the *non-I* in the borderlinking. In my interpretation, Ettinger's formulation of the *non-I* closely resembles what Lacan calls the "place of the "inter-said" [*inter-dit*], constituted by the "intra-said" [*intra-dit*] of a between-two-subjects…the very place at which the transparency of the classical subject divides" (Lacan 2006g, 677–678). But for Ettinger, the subject does not divide: the subject is a borderlinking. Additionally, for Ettinger, it is not enough to focus on the subject as divided. From a matrixial angle, we must theorize the matrixial borderlinking. This involves what she calls the "elusive feminine/prenatal incestual rapport, a lack based on its castrating foreclosure in the phallic paradigm" (Ettinger 1997, 389–390).

What Ettinger emphasizes in her theory of the matrixial is that the I of concern to the (phallic) subject emerges from "its singular *non-I*" (389). This is to say that the *I* (as individual) is never entirely separate from the m/Other and others (as *non-I*'s): all cohere in another matrixial place in time. The fact that a woman can give birth and "negotiate the unknown Other-with-in during pregnancy without psychosis, something in a Symbolic wider than the phallic-Symbolic allows them some access to this beyond/before in the matrixial stratum, even if the way it conveys meaning is yet to be discovered/invented" (388) demonstrates that there is a "bypassing-phallus sub-knowledge" (388) accompanying the I (as phallic), but also the *non-I* (as several). This axis of matrixial sub-knowledge is not only about the Other jouissance as Lacan theorizes it, but about the OSD as Ettinger develops it in her theory of the matrixial borderspace. But what else does Lacan say about the Other and does he have a theory of inter- or intra-subjectivity relevant to this other Feminine axis of difference mapped out by Ettinger?

Is the Lacanian Other a Woman?

In "The Subversion of the Subject and the Dialectic of Desire," Lacan focuses on the subject's relation to the Other's desire. It is, for him, crucial to ask in analysis: *Who is speaking?* This is because the patient's desire is in the locus of the Other. "Hence the place of the 'inter-said [*inter-dit*], constituted by the 'intra-said' [*intra-dit*] of a between-two-subjects" (Lacan 2006g, 677). When Lacan refers to the locus of the Other he is referring to the place where speech emerges. When, for example, the subject wonders who is speaking in his or her unconscious—which, for Lacan, is the Other's desire (and demand)—he or she is experiencing the "very place at which the transparency of the classical subject divides, undergoing, as it does, the effects of fading that specify the Freudian subject due to its occultation by an ever purer signifier" (677–678).

In this place of subjective division, the subject fades in its confrontation with what Lacan calls an "ever purer signifier" (678) in the orbit of the Other. The mother is, for Lacan, the first Other and where the essence of the signifier in its purity resounds. Lacan's reference to "fading" (678) involves occultation, a certain interference or eclipse of the subject, in the Imaginary, that is concordant with Ettinger's notion of fragilization (Ettinger 2009). Likewise, Ettinger's formulation of the I in the partial-subjective realm is analogous to Lacan's formulation of the I which he describes as "Being of non-being" (679). The Lacanian I is not only an effect of the signifier but "conjugated with the double aporia of a veritable subsistence" (679). The subjective junction involves a signification of the Other's desire in which the I emerges as an effect of a non-mortal death. "Being of non-being, that is how I comes on the scene as a subject who is conjugated with the double aporia of a veritable subsistence that is abolished by his knowledge, and by a discourse in which it is death that sustains existence" (679). For Lacan, procreation is tied to death and to ignore the Freudian death instinct is to misunderstand the way the signifier enables life or, in his words, the "margin beyond life that language assures" (680).

It should be remembered that when Lacan said the unconscious is structured like a language he is, in essence, suggesting that the unconscious is the Other's discourse [*discours de l'Autre*] which originates with the mother (as first and primary Other). She provides a linguistic space of subjective determination whereby the subject's own desire is set in motion by the fundamental question concerning what the Other wants from me [*Chè vuoi?*]. Another way to put this is that the Other is, for Lacan, the subject's signifying cause, thus enabling desire.

To the extent that the Lacanian subject is bound to the Other's desire and objects, and to the extent that the subject is split by the Other's discourse, this subject cannot strictly speaking be understood as One. Indeed, this subject bound to the Other is the basis upon which Ettinger will later formalize her definition of the subject-as-encounter (severality). This is also to say that Lacan's teachings lay the groundwork for her conceptualization of the matrixial borderlinking. A distinction between the two theorists may, however, be understood with respect to the fact that Lacanian analysis wishes to return to the cut of language so as to reinstate a foundational gap (in which the subject can desire and exist as separate from the m/Other), whereas Ettinger is more inclined to focus on trace-connections (as opposed to severance) as a joiner to/with/alongside the m/Other. It is not that they are two sides of the same coin but rather that they are two sides of different coins caught up in an interdependent economy of exchange involving the subject.

Of course, Ettinger is aware of the fact that Lacan's Other is not an absolute Other. Her criticism lies in the claim that Lacan does not proffer a theory of intrasubjectivity that can account for non-conscious borderlinkings and matrixial affects irreducible to signifying effects. While a full explication of the Lacan's theory of the signifier is beyond the scope of this chapter, suffice here to say that the signifier is not, for him, a mere discursive element. The subject is, for Lacan, an effect of the signifier which is not nothing. But from Ettinger's perspective, there is a corpo-Reality of the maternal body that gets reduced to nothing through Lacan's discourse, if not his theory (exactly).

For Lacan, intrasubjectivity is elaborated in relation to the signifier, which includes language and the speech of the Other. The desire of the Other of interest to Lacan is delimited by the signifier. For Lacan, the Other is ascertained by the subject as a locus of speech (Lacan 2006g, 683). The *I* and the *you* are, for Lacan, necessary for speech and speech, in turn, transforms both the *I* and the *you* in nonsymmetrical and nonreciprocal ways (Lacan 1993, 274). Much like Ettinger's partial-subjects, the *I* and the *you* of concern to Lacan are not autonomous units (individuals as such) reducible to signifiers. The desire of the Other and actual others occupying the place of *you* are central.

> In fact, the *I* is never there where it appears in the form of a particular signifier. The *I* is always there in the name of a presence that supports the discourse as a whole, whether in direct or indirect speech. The *I* is the *I* of him who is pronouncing the discourse. Underneath everything that is said there is an *I* who pronounces it. It's within this enunciation that the *you* appears (Lacan 1993, 274)…It's the *you* that says *you* in us, this *you* that always makes itself more or less discreetly heard, this *you* that speaks alone and says *You see!* To us, or, *You're always the same*. (Lacan 1993, 276)

The *you* for Lacan is always there, always accompanying the subject. This formulation of the *you* and the *I* is, in fact, a reformulation of the Freudian super-ego. Another way to put this is to say that the *you* is the Other to whom our discourse is directed as opposed to another person as such. The

Other is like the third person in a grammatical structure who does not exist. The Other is not an object or a subject who may, like the mother, go unrecognized but is the discourse supporting the subject. Lacan explains that the *you* is a "foreign body" and the signifier "pins down, quilts, the subject" (279). While the superego torments the subject Lacan explains that the *you* is also a support for the subject, however tyrannical the discourse of the Other to whom one is caused by may be in the unconscious of the subject. The important point being that the subject needs the *you* to sustain the *I*.

For Lacan, subjectivity involves a hooking function relating to the signifiers emerging from the locus of the Other. He explains: "The *you* is in the signifier what I call a way of hooking the other, of hooking him in discourse, of fastening meaning to him. It should in no way be confused with the allocator, that is, he to whom one is speaking" (299). While from a relational or, indeed, an Ettingerian perspective, the elaboration of the intrasubjective in linguistic terms may seem impersonal or lacking in its attention to affect[7] and to the body, it is intended to underscore the binding function of the signifier in both the subject and in the intersubjective realm.

Lacan also introduces what he calls "between-I's" in his seminar on the psychosis which concerns the inmixing of subjects. While Ettinger's *non-I*'s are particular to the sub-Symbolic (and not features of psychosis), Lacan explains the between-I's in relation to psychosis and insists upon their signifying structure. "As soon as there is a subject and use of the signifier, use of the between-I [*l'entre-je*] is possible, that is to say, of the interposed subject" (193). For Lacan the interposed subject is due to the fact that the Other is excluded. That is to say that the between-I phenomenon of relevance to Lacan occurs in the Imaginary register because it is predicated upon an interplay between the excluded Other and the subject. Although the between-I is imaginary and affirmed through our relations to (little) others, actual people, it is about the "subject's double, who is both his ego and not his ego" (194). The between-I is not only significant to Lacan's understanding of intersubjectivity, but to what he calls "interhuman relations" (197).

[7] See Collette Soler and Bruce Fink (2015) for a discussion of Lacan on affect.

While Ettinger's theorization of the subject-as-several is not entirely distinct from the Lacanian notion of the Other involving the I and the *you*, the Other imposed, and the place of the inter-said and the intra-said, she develops an elaborate vocabulary for theorizing what we might call Real (for her matrixial) interhuman relations. In Callum Neill's Lacanian reading of Ettinger, he notes that she gives us a way "to think the relations between I and other in a manner irreducible to consciousness, irreducible to oneness but also irreducible to separation, irreducible to isolation" (Neill 2008, 338). While Neill (2008) agrees that Ettinger's formulation of severality, involving the *I* and the *non-I*, is not dissimilar to Lacan's formulation of the non-individualized unconscious (338), he finds the vocabulary she develops for theorizing inter-subjectivity useful. In addition to developing a specialized (matrixial) vocabulary, I would add that Ettinger gives us a way to theorize an-Other sexual co-efficient relevant to the m/Other and to the Woman that has been largely overlooked in clinical applications of Lacanian theory as I will show in later chapters.

Conclusion

The Ettingerian formulation of the Woman who exists, inclusive of the Feminine and the subject-as-encounter, invite a return to Lacan. We must revisit Lacan's enigmatic sayings about the Woman who does not exist, the unconscious and the Other if we are to break new theoretical ground. Lacanian theorists have not fully articulated the clinical implications of what Lacan means when he writes that that "woman is that which has a relationship to that Other" (1998, 81). We must ask, as Ettinger does, what it means to be sexuated on the Feminine side if, as Lacan says, "Woman has a relation to the signifier of that Other…[which] remains forever Other" (81). While Ettinger does not regard this Other as an absolute Other (or limit her exposition of the subject to the signifier), she, like Lacan, maintains that there is a difference on the Feminine side worthy of investigation. This relationship to the Other is, as both Lacan and Ettinger would agree, clinically and theoretically significant.

In the next three chapters, I consider how Ettingerian theory and Lacanian theory offer different insights into the Freudian case study of

Dora, *The Ravishing of Lol Stein* by Marguerite Duras, and in Sophocles' drama *Antigone*.

Bibliography

Barnard, Suzanne. 2002. Tongues of Angels: Feminine Structure and Other Jouissance. In *Reading Seminar XX: Lacan's Major Work on Love, Knowledge, and Feminine Sexuality*, ed. Suzanne Barnard and Bruce Fink. State University of New York Press.

Bertelsen, Lone. 2004. Matrixial Refrains. *Theory, Culture & Society* 21 (1): 121–147. https://doi.org/10.1177/0263276404040484.

Brousse, Marie-Hélène. 2022. *The Feminine: A Mode of Jouissance*. Lacanian Press.

Butler, Judith. 1992. The Lesbian Phallus and the Morphological Imaginary. *Differences* 4 (1): 133–171.

Butler, Judith. 2011. *Bodies That Matter: On the Discursive Limits of Sex*. Routledge.

Cavanagh, S. L. 2016. Tiresias and psychoanalysis with/out Oedipus. European Journal of Psychoanalysis. Retrieved from http://www.journal-psycho-analysis.eu/

Cavanagh, S.L. (2018). Bracha L. Ettinger, Jacques Lacan and Tiresias: the Other Sexual Difference. Sitegeist: A Journal for Psychoanalysis and Philosophy. Issue 13. *London: The Site for Contemporary Psychoanalysis*, 32—50.

Cavanagh, S. L. 2022. "Transgender and the Other sexual difference in Vivek Shraya's Trisha." *Psychoanalysis, Culture & Society 27*: 485—501.

Copjec, Joan. 2004. *Imagine There's No Woman: Ethics and Sublimation*. The MIT Press: The MIT Press. https://doi.org/10.7551/mitpress/3668.001.0001.

Copjec, Joan. 2015. *Read My Desire: Lacan against the Historicists*, Radical Thinkers. Verso Books.

Ettinger, Bracha. 1994. The Becoming Threshold of Matrixial Borderlines. In *Travellers' Tales: Narratives of Home and Displacement*, ed. George Robertson, Melinda Mash, Lisa Tickner, Jon Bird, Barry Curtis, and Tim Putnam. Routledge.

Ettinger, Bracha. 1997. The Feminine/Prenatal Weaving in Matrixial Subjectivity-as-Encounter. *Psychoanalytic Dialogues* 7 (3): 367–405.

Ettinger, Bracha. 2000b. *Bracha Lichtenberg Ettinger: Artworking, 1985–1999*, Artworking, 1985–1999. Ludion: Palais des Beaux-Arts.

Ettinger, Bracha Lichtenberg. 2000c. Transgressing With-In-To the Feminine. In *Differential Aesthetics: Art Practices, Philosophy and Feminist Understandings*, ed. Penny Florence and Nicola Foster, 1st ed. Routledge. https://doi.org/10.4324/9781315182735-13

Ettinger, Bracha. 2001. Matrixial Gaze and Screen: Other Than Phallic and Beyond the Late Lacan. In *Bodies of Resistance: New Phenomenologies of Politics, Agency, and Culture*, ed. Laura Doyle. Northwestern University Press.

Ettinger, Bracha Lichtenberg. 2002. Trans-Subjective Transferential Borderspace. In *A Shock to Thought: Expression after Deleuze and Guattari*. Routledge.

Ettinger, Bracha. 2004. Weaving a Woman Artist With-in the Matrixial Encounter-Event. *Theory, Culture & Society* 21 (1): 69–94.

Ettinger, Bracha. 2006b. From Proto-Ethical Compassion to Responsibility: Besideness and the Three Primal Mother-Phantasies of Not-Enoughness, Devouring and Abandonment. *Athena* 1 (2): 100–135.

Ettinger, Bracha. 2006d. *The Matrixial Borderspace*, Theory out of Bounds. Vol. 28. University of Minnesota Press.

Ettinger, Bracha Lichtenberg. 2009. "Fragilization and Resistance" and "Neighborhood and Shechina". *Studies in the Maternal* 1 (2): 1–31. https://doi.org/10.16995/sim.141.

Ettinger, B. 2019. *Beyond the Death-Drive, beyond the Life-Drive: Being-toward-Birthing with Being-toward-Birth; Copoiesis and the Matrixial Eros—Metafeminist Notes*, 183–214. *Aberrant Nuptials: Deleuze and Artistic Research.*

Fink, Bruce. 2002. Knowledge and Jouissance. In *Reading Seminar XX: Lacan's Major Work on Love, Knowledge, and Feminine Sexuality*, ed. Suzanne Barnard and Bruce Fink. State University of New York Press.

Grosz, Elizabeth. 2002. *Jacques Lacan: A Feminist Introduction*. Routledge.

Grosz, Elizabeth. 2017. Psychoanalysis and the Body. In *Feminist Theory and the Body*. Routledge.

Grosz, Elizabeth. 2020a. *Sexual Subversions*. Routledge.

Grosz, Elizabeth. 2020b. *Volatile Bodies*. Routledge.

Lacan, Jacques. 1993. The Psychosis 1955—1956: The Seminar of Jacques Lacan, Book III. Edited by Jacques-Alain Miller. Translated by Russell Grigg. W.W. Norton & Company, New York and London.

Lacan, Jacques. 1997. *The Seminar of Jacques Lacan: The Psychoses 1955–1956, Book III*. Reprint edition. Translated by Jacques-Alain Miller and Russell Grigg. Norton.

Lacan, Jacques. 1998. *The Seminar of Jacques Lacan, Book XX: On Feminine Sexuality: The Limits of Love and Knowledge (Encore 1972–1973).* Edited by Jacques-Alain Miller and Bruce Fink. WW Norton & Company.

Lacan, Jacques. 2006f. Position of the Unconscious. In *Écrits: The First Complete Edition in English*, translated by Bruce Fink. W.W. Norton & Company.

Lacan, Jacques. 2006g. The Subversion of the Subject and the Dialectic of Desire in the Freudian Unconscious. In *Écrits: The First Complete Edition in English*, translated by Bruce Fink. W.W. Norton & Company.

Lacan, Jacques. 2014. *The Seminar of Jacques Lacan, Book X: Anxiety*. Edited by Jacques-Alain Miller. Translated by AR Price. Polity Press.

Morel, Geneviève. 2018. 'Feminine Conditions of Jouissance'. *In Reading Seminar XX: Lacan's Major Work on Love, Knowledge, and Feminine Sexuality*, edited by Suzanne Barnard and Bruce Fink. State University of New York Press.

Morel, Geneviève. 2002. Feminine Conditions of Jouissance. In *Reading Seminar XX: Lacan's Major Work on Love, Knowledge, and Feminine Sexuality*, ed. Suzanne Barnard and Bruce Fink. State University of New York Press.

Neill, Calum. 2008. Severality: Beyond the Compression of the Cogito. *Subjectivity* 24 (1): 325–339. https://doi.org/10.1057/sub.2008.21.

Pollock, Griselda. 2004. Thinking the Feminine: Aesthetic Practice as Introduction to Bracha Ettinger and the Concepts of Matrix and Metramorphosis. *Theory, Culture & Society (London)* 21 (1): 5–65.

Pollock, Griselda. 2007. Encounters in the Virtual Feminist Museum: Time, Space and the Archive. London; New York: Routledge.

Ragland-Sullivan, Ellie. 2012. *The Logic of Sexuation: From Aristotle to Lacan*, SUNY Series in Psychoanalysis and Culture. State University of New York Press.

Soler, Colette. 2006. *What Lacan Said about Women: A Psychoanalytic Study.* Translated by John Holland. Other Press.

Soler, Colette, and Bruce Fink. 2015. *Lacanian Affects: The Function of Affect in Lacan's Work.* Routledge.

Torre, Shanna de la. 2018. *Sex for Structuralists: The Non-Oedipal Logics of Femininity and Psychosis.* Palgrave Macmillan.

5

Dora: Hysteria and the Other Sexual Difference

Bracha L. Ettinger and Jacques Lacan offer important commentaries on the Freudian case study of Dora (Ida Bauer, 1882–1945) published in 1905. As we know from the psychoanalytic archive, Dora abruptly terminated her analysis with Freud and questions remain about how he misinterpreted her symptomatology. Both Ettinger and Lacan attend to the question of Dora's desire, to what led to the slap by the lake whereby Dora refuses the sexual proposition of Herr K. Herr K. was the husband of Dora's father's mistress, Frau K. While feminist analysis of the case is most likely to focus upon the sexual and generational boundary violations, psychoanalytic critique, including feminist psychoanalytic critique, like Ettinger's critique, focuses on questions relating to unconscious sexuality, desire, and the Feminine. Freud freely admits that Dora's desire was a mystery to him. At the time of writing the case study he thought she desired Herr K. Later he faults his own interpretation and speculates that Dora's primary interest was homosexual and focused upon Frau K. Ettinger and Lacan both build upon what Freud called a homosexual (gynophilic) current in Dora's life. Freud acknowledges his failed handling of the case and, in so doing, inaugurated over a hundred years of

S. L. Cavanagh, *Bracha L. Ettinger and Jacques Lacan*, The Palgrave Lacan Series,
https://doi.org/10.1007/978-3-032-23293-9_5

analytic speculation on Feminine sexuality and what is, not without controversy, called hysteria.[1]

In what follows I compare Ettinger's reading of the Dora case to Lacan's reading of the Dora case. I foreground their differences and points of overlap which hinge, in part, on the question of hysteria and the Feminine. I outline their points of divergence relating primarily to Dora's desire and to the way she negotiates the Feminine axis of difference theorized by Ettinger without losing track of important areas of synergy in and between her theories and those of Lacan. Both theorists agree that Freud mishandled the case and that he did not understand the central role of the Feminine in her symptomatology. Dora experienced fainting spells, depression, a variety of symptoms associated with aphonia, dyspnoea, tussis (coughing spells), and what others called unsociability. Her father insisted that his eighteen-year-old daughter see Freud after he found a suicide note. What is clear from the case is that Dora's symptoms emerged after the sexual proposition at the lake.

From Ettinger's perspective, psychoanalysis, Lacanian and otherwise, has largely ignored the woman-to-woman difference, that is the difference between the girl-becoming-woman and the woman beneath the mother. In Lacanian theory, the desire of the girl in relation to the m/Other is subsumed into the question of what the girl-becoming-woman wants from a man, thereby bypassing the Feminine dimension entirely. What Ettinger calls the daughter-mother complex is, in her view, eclipsed in Lacanian theories focused upon the phallic order of difference where the father plays a more vital role. While her critique is important, I show how Lacan did not misunderstand the relevance of Dora's desire relating not only to the Feminine but to the m/Other. As we will see in what follows, Lacan posits the question of Dora's desire in relation to the Madonna painting and in relation to hysteria. He does not sideline questions relating to feminine sexuality, as Ettinger contends, so much as he explores these questions through the discourse of the hysteric and the transference.

[1] In 1952 hysteria was removed from the Diagnostic and Statistical Manual of Mental Disorders.

Ettinger and Lacan on Dora

What Ettinger and Lacan both agree upon is that Dora's symptoms involve unconscious sexuality, but each theorist differs with respect to what her alleged hysteria means with respect to the Feminine. Lacan interprets Dora's struggle with the Feminine in terms of the hysteric's refusal to be the object cause of desire for a man. He writes that the "problem of Dora's condition is fundamentally that of accepting herself as a man's object of desire, and this is the mystery that motivates Dora's idolization of Frau K" (Lacan 2006h, 181). Ettinger, by contrast, frames Dora's struggle with the Feminine in terms of the Other Sexual Difference (OSD) whereby she is not interested in the man (or the phallus-as-signifier) but in a woman-to-woman difference. Dora was estranged from her mother, her aunt died, and she, in Ettinger's reading, adored Frau K. because she was a mother-like figure (until, of course, Frau K. betrays her by siding with her husband in the troubling scene by the lake). From the matrixial angle, Dora's question is not about sexual positioning as masculine or feminine, but about the status of the Feminine in the Symbolic which, as Lacan agrees, eclipses elements of the woman's being.

Lacan knew that Freud should not have stopped asking questions about Dora's desire. Instead of posing questions enabling Dora to elaborate upon her own desire, as related to the Feminine, Freud *gave* her answers which, of course, say more about his own countertransference than anything of relevance to Dora. Lacan also recognized, like Ettinger, the significance of the Madonna painting to Dora (to which I will return), and how her question was not about sexual positioning, but about the status of the Feminine and what it means to be a woman. In Lacanian theory, the hysteric is curious about how elements of the woman's being exist without a symbol. As we know from his discussion of the four discourses in Seminar XVII, the discourse of the hysteric is epistemological, as opposed to pathological. Lacan situates Dora's question in relation to the hysteric's discourse, which addresses the master from her position as barred subject. This is an important discourse in the Lacanian paradigm that generates knowledge, but for Ettinger, hysteria is a mode of questioning that becomes symptomatic when access to the matrixial is blocked. This is to say that hysteria is not really a discourse in the Ettingerian frame so much as it is an indication of how the woman-to-woman difference involving the girl-daughter and the m/Other is foreclosed.

Lacan agrees that there is something of significance relevant to hysteria in women as exemplified in the case of Dora that needs to be explicated from what he calls the "ladies' side." He tries to analyze this in relation to the Freudian case of the "female homosexual" (Freud, 1963) who, like Dora, was caught up in a humiliating drama relating, in part, to her father's gaze. The homosexual woman was nineteen at the time of her analysis and was, like Dora, referred to Freud by her father. While Dora ended her analysis with Freud, the homosexual woman's treatment was ended prematurely by Freud, allegedly, because of *her* negative transference which, from the perspective of the present, can more obviously be seen as Freud's inability to handle the transferential dynamics.

In his seminar on anguish (*angoisse*), Lacan sets up a comparison between Dora's aphonia and the homosexual woman's impaired mobility; the latter was walking with her lover at the time she was caught by her father's formidable gaze. Both are, in different ways, reduced to what Lacan calls the object-cause of desire (*object a*) for the man. In seminar X, Lacan describes the homosexual woman's act (relating to a suicide attempt) as an attempt to leave the scene in which she is bound to her father's desire and to his law involving, among other things, a totalizing identification with the *object a*. Lacan says, "What comes at this moment to the subject [the homosexual woman], is her absolute identification to this *a* [object causing the father's desire], to which she is reduced. Confrontation with this desire of the father upon which all her behaviour is constructed, with this law which is presentified in the look of the father, it is through this that she feels herself identified and at the same moment, rejected, ejected off the stage" (Lacan 2011, 99)

From Lacan's perspective, the homosexual woman, like Dora, is, through her symptomology, but also through her refusal to be a pond, or object, in her father's fantasy formation, attempting to free herself from a sexual positioning in which she does not exist, at least not fully, in the man's libidinal economy. In his essay "Guiding Remarks for a Conversation on Female Sexuality," Lacan does not deny, but insists upon the centrality of the Feminine in female homosexuality. He states: "in all forms of female homosexuality, even unconscious, the supreme interest is in femininity" (Lacan 2006e, 619). Lacan, like Ettinger, agrees that there is something relating to the Feminine that is evacuated in the Symbolic, but also in phallic jouissance. But Ettinger is less concerned about who the woman is for the man and more concerned about who the girl-(daughter)-becoming-woman is for another woman or m/Other.

It is important to note that Ettinger does not use the Freudian case of the homosexual woman to establish a point of reference for Dora, but a fictional character, Lol Stein, in the Marguerite Duras (1966) novel which I discuss in the following chapter. Although Ettinger writes about Dora and Lol Stein together, I focus on the OSD as relevant to Dora in this chapter.

The Other Sexual Difference

What Ettinger calls an "originary difference of the feminine" (2006, 70) is of paramount concern to Dora. For everyone, the first axis of sexual difference pivots around an adult-female as m/Other. Ettinger explains that this difference is not to be understood in terms of phallic cuts and oppositions, but in relation to *a-links*, traces, and resemblances. We are like and non-like others in the matrixial sphere. But the likeness is of particular relevance to the female-girl-daughter because she is more like the female-woman-m/Other in anatomical form than the male-boy-son. In Ettinger's interpretation, Dora is not concerned with the primal scene of sexual intercourse between parents (or adult substitutes), but with the primal scene of birth inclusive of what it means to become a woman in-relation-to-the-m/Other. The problem, as Ettinger defines it, is that Freud was focused on Oedipal sexuality without understanding that Dora was searching for a matrixial encounter with an adult woman. She had to work through the OSD that would enable her to transition from girl to woman and potential m/Other. As discussed in previous chapters, regardless of gender, trans- or cisgender status, and natal sex, each becoming-subject first differentiates themselves from the m/Other-woman in the Ettingerian account. The OSD is about a matrixial-transformative sexual move concerning a maternal figure. It is an axis of Feminine difference that comes before Oedipal sexuality from a developmental viewpoint and occurs alongside the Oedipal from a structural viewpoint, but is altogether different. It is also, as Ettinger argues, distinct from masculine and feminine sexual positioning in the Lacanian model of sexuation. The OSD concerns life, Eros, and the "riddle of the desirability-in-itself that emanates from the Other-woman" (63).

Questions about Feminine desire and the Other-woman-m/Other are not sidelined in Ettinger's theory of the OSD. Dora was, for Ettinger, desiring to "emerge into becoming-with-an-other" (65). The matrixial co-emergence of concern to Ettinger is an affective and aesthetic resonance field that she likens to a shared psychic cloth.[2] Dora circles back to scenes of desire felt to be primal because she is longing to be fascinating, and to be fascinated by, an older woman-m/Other. Ettinger explains that Dora's mother did not fulfill her daughter's longing to be seen and desired. Let us remember that the mystery of desire first concerns the woman-m/Other in Ettingerian psychoanalysis. Mysteries and enigmas of femininity and desirability need to be negotiated before Dora can become a woman. Ettinger contends that a girl cannot become a woman without working through a woman-to-woman matrixial difference. The girl-daughter "looks for a Woman-Mother figure whom she might adore and whose secrets she would be able to share on condition that such a m/Other would open herself to allow such a sharing and accommodate her gaze" (67). Without a desiring matrixial gaze can the girl become a desiring subject in her own rite, find desire in and about other women (irreducible to lesbian sexuality), and care for girls-becoming-women in a matrixial alliance? Ettinger thinks not. But it is not enough for the m/Other to desire the girl and share in the enigma of femininity, the daughter-becoming-woman must access something of what Ettinger describes as the "ravishing m/Other-Thing-Event in-itself as becoming with-in encounter" (68).

[2] Ettinger's notion of the shared or "common cloth" (2006, 75) is a matrixial variant of the Lacanian plait which he explicates in his seminars on *The Sinthome* (1975–1976) and *Les non-dupes errent* (1973–1974). The Lacanian plait, which is a braid involving the Real, the Imaginary, and the Symbolic, particular to each individual-subject is, in Ettinger's matrixial variation, modified to denote the trans-subjective sphere (2006, 80–81). Ettinger also refers to the psychic cloth as an "interweaving" and as a "matrixial fabric" (2006, 77).

The m/Other-Thing-Event involves an encounter that is, for Ettinger, distinguishable from the signifying cut in the Lacanian frame. It is an encounter that is, as I discuss in Chap. 7, comparable to the blinding splendor of Antigone, as Lacan phrases it in his Seminar on Ethics. It is also, as both Ettinger and Lacan would agree, jouissant. For Ettinger, "blind desirability" (68) is both fatal and ravishing. Ettinger elaborates upon the m/Other-Event-Encounter as occurring in a matrixial sphere of unconscious severality. Recall that the Ettingerian subject is not individual, but more than one. The co-emergence between the girl-becoming-woman and a m/Other (as *non-I*) is a borderlinking that needs time to coalesce; it is fundamental to the matrixial alliance. Ettinger explains that "Subjectivity-as-encounter emerges, where the Other-mother is never an absolute Other, absolutely separate, and where the first difference for a woman (a female child) is from another woman (a female grown-up)" (79).

The m/Other-Thing-Event for Dora was brought to an abrupt halt by the sexual proposition at the lake, a proposition precipitating a slap. Dora was devastated not only by Herr K.'s sexual provocation, but by his confession: My wife means nothing to me. Dora needed and valued the Other woman (Herr K.'s wife) as partner-in-difference on the way to becoming woman. What enrages Dora and leads to the now famous slap is not only the adulterous seduction attempt, but the audacity of Herr K. to say that his wife, who adopts a maternal role for Dora, means nothing to him.

Let us remember that for Lacan, the Woman does not exist. But from an Ettingerian perspective, the m/Other-beneath-the-woman is all important. While Frau K is not Dora's mother, she represents the woman beneath the m/Other. For Dora, the m/Other is "always almost lost and longed-for and almost always not-yet found again, both outside (in reality) and inside the self (in phantasm), who shines through another woman who is relating to a man to whom the subject intimately relates as well" (Ettinger 2006, 68). Dora longs to be included in the rapturous scene involving her father and Herr K., but not to the exclusion of Frau K. This is not superfluous, but central to working through a primary matrixial sexual difference.

Ettinger posits a primary sexual difference between the girl-child and the m/Other which also concerns the boy-child's sexual difference form the m/Other, but in a different way. What the case study of Dora so beautifully illustrates from a matrixial point of view is that the OSD "produces for men and women a different, non-Oedipal sublimation where, in the search for *non-I*(s), the *jouissance* is of the borderlinking itself" (Ettinger 2001, 110). This is to say that of primary concern to the becoming-subject and perhaps, even more significant to the girl-daughter, is the borderlinking with the m/Other and/or Other Woman. "To establish a borderlink while differentiating oneself from the other is a pathway to the Other that transgresses individual limits" (Ettinger 2006, 80). This borderlinking in the matrixial is of great importance to Feminine sexuality.

Consider that borderlinking is metramorphic, as discussed in Chap. 2, and driven by a Feminine Eros relevant to the *a-link* (a matrixial variant on Lacan's *object a*). It is also, as Ettinger explains, an encounter-event in the Real at the basis of the OSD. The metramorphosis is about asymmetrical co-emergence in, with and alongside Others in a shared matrixial covenant that borrows something, in the Ettingerian elaboration, from the Deleuzian and Guattarian notion of becoming and assemblage. But what is of paramount significance, in the Ettingerian account, is that there is, as has already been stated, an Other non-Oedipal axis of sexual difference involving the m/Other. Not only does Ettinger's theory of the OSD displace the primary importance of the father in the Oedipal story authored by Freud and the central importance of the phallic signifier in the teachings of Lacan, but also it gives us another way to understand the symptomatology of the girl-daughter along with the hysteric.

The Hysteric

Much has been written on the question of hysteria in psychoanalysis and in culture at large, on the sexism built into the diagnostic, and the way it has been used to render female bodies pathological (Gilman et al. 2022, and Showalter 1985). For those unfamiliar with Lacanian writing on hysteria, it is important to know that he does not pathologize what he calls the structure of hysteria. As noted above, Lacan focuses on the discourse of the hysteric and the way it generates knowledge central to psychoanalysis. For Ettinger, hysteria is a response to something relating to the daughter-m/Other borderlinking that is interrupted or blocked.

Lacan and Ettinger agree that those designated hysteric are bound by a question concerning sexuality, but they differ with respect to the place of the Woman in the question. For Lacan, the hysteric does not want to become a Woman (as sexuated subject). In other words, she does not want to be the object cause of the man's desire. For Ettinger, the hysteric is not primarily concerned with what it means to be a Woman in relation to a man, but in relation to the m/Other. From a matrixial perspective, Dora is not undecided about becoming a woman, but struggling to become a Woman because something relating to the borderlinking with her mother has been severed. Recall that the Ettingerian Woman is not a sexuated subject, but a Real non-linguistic predicate for borderlinkings in the matrixial. As discussed in Chap. 4, the Woman is a transitive condition of co-emerge between the subject and their Others (*non-I's*). Dora is abandoned by her mother who would, typically, enable a metramorphic borderlinking. Let us also remember that Dora's actual mother is unavailable, depressed and, apparently, disinterested in Dora-as-daughter. The Other woman, Frau K., is, like her own mother, devalued by her husband. More than this, Frau K., as maternal stand-in, sides with her husband, Herr K., against Dora in the final account. For Dora, the question is not *Am I a man or a woman, and what is the difference?*, but rather: *What is the difference between me and the m/Other woman who is devalued?*

Both Ettinger and Lacan agree that the m/Other is central to the girl/hysteric's question about desire. In the Lacanian view, every subject's question is about *what* or *whom I am to you*. For Ettinger, the question to the m/Other posed by the girl-daughter is more specific. She poses her question to "another woman-m/Other-Encounter, to a subject conceived as alike-non-same, from whom one is differentiating-in-joining and from whom one in severality can open a distance but only in proximity" (2006, 184). Boy-sons may do the same, but in Ettinger's view, the physical likeness between the girl-daughter and the mother, Real and imagined, is sexually differentiated.

While the emphasis Ettinger puts on the m/Other is important, it does not contradict the Lacanian claim that the unconscious is trans-individual. If we listen carefully to the hysteric, we can hear that they are not (only) asking if they are a man or a woman but rather if they are one or two (or more). While this question is, for Ettinger, about the structure of severality in the matrixial, it is, for Lacan, central to the hysteric's discourse (whereby the agent of the address speaks from their position as divided subject). Lacan contends that the true hysterical question is not "*Am I a man or a woman*?" but rather is "*Is there One or not?*" (Lacan 38, 102, emphasis added). The question of the One is not, in my view, unlike the matrixial question relating to the Woman in the borderlinking. Both questions engage the presence and status of an Other in the orbit of the I. Both psychoanalysts agree that the first Other is the mother. But Ettinger stresses the central importance of the Other matrixial difference involving the mother to the girl-daughter, whereas Lacan focuses on the sexuating coefficient. Let us now turn to the Madonna to better understand what Ettinger calls the "Girl-to-m/Other" sexual difference.

The Madonna

Like Lacan, Ettinger attends to the way Dora was transfixed by the Sistine Madonna in the Dresden Gallery. When Freud asks Dora what interests her about the Madonna she answers, as if to accentuate the obvious, "the Madonna" (Freud 1963, 96). Dora stared at the Madonna for two hours, "rapt in silent admiration" (Ettinger 2006, 60), but Freud did not pursue the question of the Madonna from what Ettinger calls a matrixial angle. Instead, his analysis of the case hovers around what Dora wants from a man, whether this man may be Herr K., her father or, in fact, Freud the psychoanalyst himself. In Ettinger's critique of the Freudian case, she contends that Dora leaves Freud because he does not understand the "Girl-to-m/Other" difference of relevance to her struggle. In other words, he neglects the non-Oedipal woman-to-woman matrixial relation of centrality to the Dora case.

It is not a credit to Freud that he neglected the m/Other in his clinical work with Dora. As evident in the case study, he focuses on the father, wonders what Dora wants from a man and then, long after the analysis has been terminated (by Dora), he wonders what she wants from a woman but in Oedipal terms. This is to say that he wonders if her desire is homosexual and directed toward Frau K. Ettinger argues that matrixial desire, as explained in previous chapters, is not reducible to sexual orientation because it is not phallic. Dora's desire is not genital, but matrixial. As Ettinger explains, Dora's intrigue with the Madonna and Frau K. was not an expression of lesbian desire. Her desire was matrixial (non-Oedipal).

> She desired to be caught in a move of fascination that belongs to femininity, a move composed of a fascination of a girl toward a woman-mother figure, who is fascinated too by the daughter-girl and who allows her sufficient proximity to sustain the illusion of inclusion in her mature elusive femininity – a femininity which is not directed at the girl but outside and away from her. (Ettinger 2006, 62)

As we know from the case, Dora witnessed a series of failed and abandoned relations with older women. Her mother ignored and rejected her, her aunt (who initiated sex education) died, and she was betrayed by her father's lover Frau K. Ettinger's suggestion is that Dora turned to a painting of the Madonna when no adult women were there to enable a metramorphic event whereby she could leave the position of girl-daughter to become a woman. "So she leaned on what cannot betray or die: an object of art that corresponds to the internal subjective-object of her phantasm" (62). Her phantasy was that the Madonna was looking back at her, was fascinated by her, and enabling a transformation of matrixial links and imprints relevant to the OSD.

Dora's fascination with the Madonna illustrates the importance of the m/Other to the OSD, an axis of sexual difference that predates and is irreducible to the Oedipal sexual difference of concern to Freud. In Ettinger's interpretation, Dora was raptured by the Madonna because she was waiting for a transformation in the matrixial borderlinking whereby she could be seen by an older woman as maternal stand-in. "Dora created a moment of looking at the Madonna's painting as a matrixial encounter-event by her unconscious urge to produce transformation in the traces of imprints of earlier moments of encounter that had failed" (61). Ettinger is not suggesting that Dora does not become a woman in gendered terms, but rather that there is something from the perspective of the matrixial that does not complete a progression. "Even when she became a woman, a wife, and a mother, she remained a girl along the feminine-matrixial differential axis, unable to close the gap between these two poles: the girl's and the woman's" (63). Ettinger's interest in the Dora case is not about her (phallic) sexuality, but about the OSD in which she remains a girl in what she calls the "woman-to-woman differential string" (63).

For Ettinger, this woman-to-woman differential string is what Freud could not understand and thus interpret. Because the girl-daughter is more like the woman-m/Other in anatomical form and reproductive capacity, there is more at stake in her differentiation from the woman-m/Other than there is for the boy-son. This is what Ettinger claims Freud misses in his analysis of Dora and she is right. In retrospect, we can see how Freud does not pay sufficient attention to the adult women in Dora's life including but not limited to the mother. Given that Dora had a hysterical attack of appendicitis, high-fever, abdominal and violent menstrual pain after her aunt's death, it is also curious that Freud fails to acknowledge the centrally important role of the aunt in Dora's life-history. In the Ettingerian interpretation, Dora is not only raptured by the question of the Feminine in matrixial terms but also attuned to her mother's non-presence (or marginalization) in the family drama.

The hysteric's physical ailments may, as feminist psychoanalytic theorists note, map the complexities of the maternal discourse or what Ettinger might call, along with Abraham and Torok (1994), the transgenerational phantom-like trace of an Other's suffering through psychosomatic symptomology (Cavanagh 2018a). Ettinger's work prompts us to consider how hysterics may identify with a discontent born of the m/Other's non-presence in the Symbolic. For the hysteric, there may be an acute awareness of how the maternal-Feminine is eclipsed in the Symbolic circuit. This is a vitally important line of inquiry that needs to be further explored from a feminist psychoanalytic angle.

But let us return to Ettinger's critical intervention. Thus far, she claims that there is a difference between the woman-to-woman difference, of relevance to Dora, and Oedipal sexual difference. Second, she reminds us that this woman-to-woman difference is not reducible to gender identity, sexual orientation or sexual positioning (masculine or feminine sexuation). Dora is not "exploring the enigma of the woman as a desired *object* for the man, neither as a lost or missing nor as a present object – the cause of the man's (or the father's) desire" (Ettinger 2006, 63). Dora is, for Ettinger, negotiating the OSD which predates, yet occurs alongside, phallic sexuality. Desire, in matrixial terms, is about borderlinking and a "vanishing and fading, but never disappearing link" that is transformative and particular to the Feminine axis of difference. For Ettinger, the OSD involves the riddle and enigma of "desirability-in-itself that emanates from the Other-woman" (63).

In the Madonna, Dora was searching for archaic matrixial traces, affective links, and an out-of-time encounter event with the woman-m/Other; an encounter that Ettinger describes as enigmatic.

> This is the enigma of the closeness and distance, resemblance in difference of the girl from the blinding and stupefying ravishing *Woman-m/Other-in-encounter*, considered archaic in that both herself and the encounter belong to the remarkable matrixial time-out-of-time and matrixial border-space, and in that the *Woman-m/Other with-in the encounter* is neither present nor lost, neither assimilated nor rejected by the emerging self. (Ettinger 2006, 64)

We might say that the ravishing encounter-event with the Woman-m/Other is Real in Lacanian terms, but for Ettinger, it involves fascinance.

As Ettinger (2006) explains in her discussion of fascinance, matrixial encounter-events involve differentiation and appear as apparitions. In the girl-daughter and m/Other matrixial relation, partial-subjects (*non-I*'s) are affected by "rare apparitions of fascinating scenes in reality" (2006, 64). From a Lacanian perspective, we might say that fascinance involves the gaze of the Other, jouissance, and phantasy. But for Ettinger, fascinance is specific to the matrixial borderspace. In her interpretation, Dora longs to be caught in a desiring gaze in/by/with an Other older woman (as maternal subject) to enable a matrixial transition to womanhood. As Ettinger further explains, Dora "desired to be caught in a move of fascination that belongs to femininity, a move composed of a fascination of a girl toward a woman-mother figure, who is fascinated too by the daughter-girl and who allows her sufficient proximity to sustain the illusion of inclusion in her mature elusive femininity – a femininity which is not directed at the girl but outside and away from her" (2006, 62).

In Ettingerian psychoanalysis, fascinance is an ethical acknowledgment of the Real as it affects others. She defines it as an "aesthetic affect that operates in the suspension and generous prolongation of the duration of encounter-event" (2009, 3). It is proto-ethical and occurs along what Ettinger calls "trans-sensuous strings" (3). Fascinance is a matrixial variant on fascinum (which appears in Lacan's writings), the latter of which is, in Ettinger's view, fetishistic and freezes the subject in the gaze of the onlooker. Ettinger's writing on Dora (and Lol Stein which I discuss in the following chapter) underscores the difficulties involved in the process of becoming a woman when there is a lack of fascinance. Dora is, as Ettinger explains, raptured by the question of how one becomes a Woman, with what it is to be in a matrixial covenant and to desire as a woman. What sets off a hysterical response is the fact that her yearning to be recognized by an Other older woman remains in abeyance. The position of the hysteric gains currency within the domain of phallic sexual difference when Feminine difference lacks inscription. Hysteria is, for Ettinger, a "subjectivizing response on the part of women to men's definition of female sexuality" (2006, 184). It occurs, as noted above, when one's access to the matrixial is blocked.

What Dora waits to see in the Madonna is not an image-as-object but a matrixial encounter-event that would enable her to make a passage from girl-to-woman. As Ettinger explains in relation to Lol Stein, "If the image is sustained long enough, and the gesture of the scene is completed, the distance between the Girl and the Woman will fade out, Girl and Woman will become sisters in the feminine" (2006, 65). Speaking specifically about the fictional character Lol Stein in the novel by Marguerite Duras (1964), Ettinger concludes that "[Lol Stein] wanted to be co-re-born as a woman in relations of fascination" (2006, 85). The Feminine re-birth occurs by and through a compassionate gaze, one that enables the girl to be held in a nurturing look long enough to complete the transition into a "woman." Dora's search for a woman-beneath-the-m/Other to return her fascination and thus to be fascinated by her, as a girl-becoming-a-woman, was repeatedly disappointed. As Ettinger puts it, Dora is "*prematurely evacuated*" from the "m/Other-Event-Encounter" (68, emphasis in original).

How might we interpret this premature evacuation in Lacanian terms and does Lacan's writing on hysteria and the transference neglect the m/Other?

The Transference and Hysteria

In his "Presentation on Transference," Lacan critiques Freud's mishandling of the transference in the Dora case. In the presentation Lacan gave in 1951 at the Romance Language-Speaking Psychoanalysts, he underscores the damaging effects of the analysts' resistance in the countertransference. Lacan says that what is said to be "negative on the part of the subject [is] the doing [*opération*] of the analyst who interprets it" (Lacan 2006h, 178). This is to say that the only resistance in psychoanalysis is, for Lacan, to be found in the analyst. In Lacan's reading, Freud over identifies with Herr K. and misses the significance of Frau K. As a result, Freud fails to grasp the function of the quadrille (Dora, her father and the K.'s) and its relevance to hysteria. Lacan believes that Freud should have focused the analysis on questions relating to what Frau K. meant to Dora as opposed to inserting his own identificatory interest in Herr K. as the solution Dora resisted. It is not, as Freud later thought, that he neglected Dora's latent homosexuality, but that his bias lay in the presumptive importance of the paternal figure at the expense of the mother.

> I would say that this has to be ascribed to a bias, the very same bias that falsifies the conception of the Oedipus complex right from the outset, making him consider the predominance of the paternal figure to be natural, rather than normative --- the same bias that is expressed simply in the well-known refrain, "Thread is to needle as girl is to boy." (182)

Like Ettinger, Lacan is critical of sexism and normativity in Freudian psychoanalysis. It is also interesting to note that Lacan sides with Ernest Jones who contends that female homosexuality, latent and manifest, is about "the supreme interest…in femininity" (Lacan 2006e, 619). This supreme interest concerns the mother or her substitute, and not the father or heterosexuality configured in Oedipal and phallic terms. The man, when he plays a part in the fantasy, is an "invisible witness…[to] the care taken by the [female] subject in giving her partner jouissance" (619).

This suggests that Lacan was aware of the central importance of the Feminine in the Dora case, even as he approaches the Feminine through what Ettinger calls a phallic angle. For Lacan, Dora is not (only) used by Herr K. *She* instrumentalizes *him*: "Dora in fact uses Herr K. as her ego, in that it is by means of him that she is effectively able to support her relationship with Frau K" (Lacan 1997, 91). Lacan describes Herr K. as a "mediating fourth person" (91), much like the invisible witness identified by Jones. Lacan does not suppose that Dora's interest in Frau K. is about same-sex attraction. Rather, for him, it is about a rivalrous identification with Dora's father. Lacan makes more of the fact that Dora's mother is, in his words, "obliterated in the parental couple" (91), than Freud does. In the Freudian case, the mother is described as an "uncultivated woman and above all a foolish [woman]" (Freud 1963, 13). Dora, in Freud's interpretation, does not hold her mother in high esteem. Unfortunately, Lacan does not elaborate upon what the obliteration of the mother-wife from the parental couple means for Dora. He only says that the triangle, involving Dora and her parents, became unbearable for her.

In Lacan's interpretation, Dora is concerned about what it means to be a woman and thus to be without a signifier for her sex as such. Dora uses Herr K. as an imaginary penis-instrument (or signifying prosthetic) to apprehend what she cannot symbolize (Lacan 1997, 178). Lacan reasons that there are more female hysterics than male hysterics because it is so difficult to symbolize woman's sex. Female hysterics wonder about what it means to be a woman but do not become women. This is not a pathology so much as it is, as Lacan speculates in his Seminar on the Psychosis (178), a way of identifying with the father or, as he contends in his later work, identifying with the man's symptom.

While Dora was interested in what it is about Frau K. that her father desires, what it is that he loves in her beyond Dora herself (as daughter) alongside her own mother, the thing she "latches on to is this something that is loved by her father in another, in so far as she doesn't know what it is" (Lacan 2020, 133). In reference to Dora, Lacan asks "Where does she end up in fact, if not confronted by a fundamental question on the subject of her sex? Not on what sex she is, but *What is it to be a woman*?" (1997, 171). Lacan notes that both boy-son and girl-daughter wonder what it is to be a woman, but their sexual explorations take distinct paths. "For the woman, the realization of her sex is not accomplished in the Oedipus complex in a way symmetrical to that of the man's, not by identification with the mother, but on the contrary by identification with the paternal object, which assigns her an extra detour" (172).

While Ettinger brings the m/Other into the equation more fully than does Lacan, both she and Lacan foreground the role of the Other woman in the case study. Moreover, Lacan knows, like Ettinger, that the hysteric's interest concerns the Feminine. For Lacan, the female-hysteric does not become a woman but explores the question of femininity from the sidelines. She does not wish to partake in the sexual non-rapport but to signify something about the impasse from the woman's side through her symptomatology.

Dora, like all hysterics in the Lacanian frame, enjoys through privation. This is accomplished through substitution: your desire is my desire. The interest the hysteric takes in the Other's desire, or in the way the Other lacks (or suffers), is not sacrificial so much as it is a defense against the Other's jouissance. In *Seminar XX*, Lacan (1998) explains that the hysteric wants to be the signifier of the Other's desire as distinct from the object of the man's satisfaction. To be the signifier of the Other's desire, that is to say the phallus in Lacanian terms, is not to be a man exactly, but to be what the Other desires. It is through this being by proxy that the hysteric, in this case Dora, explores the enigma of the Feminine involving, but not limited to, what it means to be a woman. For Lacan, the hysteric cultivates a fantasy whereby she is, or becomes, what the Other does not have. What differentiates the female-hysteric from the woman, in the Lacanian interpretation, is the fact that the former needs to excavate a lack in the Other whereas the latter does not.

It is curious that Ettinger does not acknowledge Lacan's interest, however incompletely elaborated, in the Feminine and the Other, of significance to Dora. His writing on hysteria and the transference are attempts, in my reading, to articulate what Ettinger calls an OSD irreducible to object choice. Where Lacan addresses an irresponsible handling of the transference on Freud's part (and Ettinger would no doubt agree on this score), Ettinger posits a theory of transitivism to grasp the subject-hysteric's relation to the Other.

Transitivism

In Ettingerian theory, transitivism (the *I* with the Other as *non-I*) is central to the OSD as discussed in Chap. 3. In most psychoanalytic theories, transitivism is viewed as regressive and infantile. But for Ettinger transitivism is a Feminine sexual difference. There is, as Ettinger laments, a way that the Feminine is, in most psychoanalytic writing, dismissed as symbiotic, characterized by fusion or, at worst, psychotic. For Lacan, transitivism is connected to the formation of the ego and involves a process whereby the child-subject is fixated upon an alienating image in the form of another child-subject (likening it to the mirror stage). But transitivism, for Ettinger, is a Feminine difference central to the subject-as-several. It is phantasmatic, jouissant and Real. It is also not something one outgrows, although Feminine transitivity lacks phallic inscription. While Ettinger's interpretation of transitivism differs from Lacan's interpretation of transitivism, he, like Ettinger, agrees that it is erotic. He explains that in the transitive "erotic relationship, in which the human individual fixates on an image that alienates him from himself, that we find the energy and the form from which the organization of the passions that he [the subject] will call his ego originates" (2006j, 113).

Where a critical difference lies is in their theorization of transitivity as it relates to subjectivity. Ettinger contends that the Feminine transitive relation is fortifying, whereas Lacan emphasizes aggressivity in the transitive object relation. It is worth noting that for Ettinger there is no aggressivity in the matrixial. There is trauma and destructive deposits of jouissance when access to the matrixial is blocked or torn (as I will further discuss in the final chapter on Antigone), but the transitive Feminine relation is not destructive. For Lacan, by contrast, there is narcissism in the transitive identification. The ego, as Lacan understands it, is constituted by a relation of alienation in the mirror stage and aggressivity in the orbit of the Other. The ego is, in other words, an Other that "sets itself up in a duality internal to the subject" (93). Another way to put this is that where Ettinger foregrounds Eros in the borderlinking with the Other (as *non-I*), Lacan views the subject's egoist relation to the Other as fractious. As he contends in his seminar on *The Psychosis*:

> In every relationship with the other, even an erotic one, there is some echo of this relation of exclusion, *it's either him or me*, because, on the imaginary plane, the human subject is so constituted that the other is always on the point of re-adopting the place of mastery in relation to him, because there is an ego in him that is always in part foreign to him, a master implanted in him over and above his set of tendencies, conduct, instincts, and drives. (93)

This is Lacan's way of saying that the ego and the drives are in conflict. Any "imaginary equilibrium with the other always bears the mark of a fundamental instability" (93).

For Ettinger, there seems to be equanimity in and between partial-subjects in the matrixial transitive encounter. But in the Lacanian interpretation, we may find aggression in the way Dora tries to usurp the position of the mother/Other woman. Lacan explains that Dora projects herself into the position of Frau K. because she is, as her father's mistress, what is loved by her father beyond her. "Frau K. is the living incarnation of what Dora can neither know nor cognize in this situation, where she finds nowhere to accommodate herself. When it comes to love, someone is loved over and above what that someone is. Ultimately it's something this someone is lacking, whoever they are" (Lacan 2020, 134).

Dora positions herself between the lovers, her father, and Frau K. So long as she is included in the dyad, as a third, she is happy. But there is also a fourth figure: Herr K. Lacan refers to the broken bonds in the quadrille in ways that are not dissimilar to the way Ettinger speaks about tears in the matrixial web. The bonds are described by Lacan as "subtle and ambiguous but which in each case carry a meaning and are perfectly oriented" (136). They are not unlike the affective trace-connections, *a-links*, and strings of concern to Ettinger in matrixial webs. Herr K., like Frau K., but in a different way, was like the fourth (sinthomatic) ring (or string in Ettingerian terms) holding the family together. Lacan seems to suggest that the "four-fold group composition" (1997, 91) was necessary and that until the fateful day at the lake she "behaved admirably in order to avoid any scenes and to ensure that her father had normal relations with the woman" (9). Dora's slap and refusal of what is seen, from the perspective of the present, to be an indecent proposal disturbs what Lacan calls the "equilibrium of the situation" (91). Lacan compares the impropriety to nothing beyond what we might see in a Viennese operetta (91). He presumes that Dora was comfortable with the situation until the foursome was in danger of collapsing because it is after the day at the lake, when she rejects Herr K., that her symptoms, including aphonia, become pronounced and she accuses her father of prostituting her in an inappropriate exchange.

Hysteria and the Odious Exchange

Lacan refers to the way Dora is subject to an "odious exchange" by her father who seems to offer his daughter up "defenseless to Herr K's attentions" (2006h, 178). He also says that Dora's father "turns a blind eye" (178). The father knows but will not see the way he has made his daughter into an object of circulation and substitution. The quadrille is what Lacan attends to in his discussion of the exchange of goods, an exchange which is not wholly distinct from the erotic and aesthetic bonds between partners-in-difference in the matrixial webs of concern to Ettinger. Lacan refers to the circulation of "precious gifts" (179) in the foursome. He follows the links between what he also calls "parallel gifts" through an economy of exchange that functions like the meanderings of the signifier. Lacan does not reduce the quadrille to a unit of signification but explicates the process through which Herr K.'s wife is "reduced here to this lateral link in the chain of exchanges" (179).

Lacan believes, like Freud, that Dora gets something from the minuet of four actors, specifically an object: Frau K. While Ettinger does not explicate Dora's relationship to Frau K. in the language of objects, but rather in the language of links (as in *a-links*), their assessments of the mystery and enigma of femininity rapturing Dora are not dissimilar.

Lacan first refers to Frau K. as an object for Dora and then says "Frau K is not an individual, but a mystery, the mystery of Dora's own femininity, by which I mean her bodily femininity" (180).

In Lacan's assessment, Dora, like all hysterics, struggles to "assume [*assumer*] her own body" (181) which is what gives way to conversion symptoms. Although Lacan is in agreement with Freud that Dora is only "a little hysteric; she doesn't have many symptoms" (1997, 91), there is, in his interpretation, an association of Woman with a "primitive oral desire" (2006h, 180) evident not only in her aphonia but in her "unusual object relationships" (1997, 90). These unusual object relations are not about female homosexuality, but about Dora's refusal to be an object of desire for the man. What is an ever-present question in clinical work with hysterics is who their "love object really is" (90). For Lacan, Dora has access to Frau K. through an identification with Herr K. (the masculine partner), but what she wants from Frau K. is not reducible to sex. She is interested in what a man desires in Frau K. as a woman. There is, as Lacan argues, no signifier for sexual difference in the unconscious. Dora palliates the lack of a signifier for the Woman through an identification with Herr K. (on the imaginary level) and her father (on the symbolic level). In Véronique Voruz's Lacanian reading, "It is when she [Dora] is confronted with the real of a sexual demand that she is brought back to her own jouissance, which was until then comfortably channeled by the dynamics of her identifications" (2007, 163). Dora's anxiety (*angoisse*) is precipitated by the way she, as opposed to Frau K., is desired by Herr K. The question of her sexual positioning can no longer be kept in abeyance. Dora is confronted with the jouissance of the Other (Herr K.) without the mediating support of a fantasy involving, among other things, her identifications with the desire of the men and Frau K (as object).

In *Encore*, Lacan explains that the hysteric's fantasy, which acts to mediate the Other's jouissance and related questions about what it means to be a woman, involves the father's desire (1998, 368). Her Real identification is with the object desired by the Other, which is the Woman. What is significant about female-hysteria in the Lacanian frame is the interposing role of other women at the level of fantasy. This role comes at the expense of alienation because Dora does not enable herself to be an object-subject of the Other's love. This is not to suggest that Dora should have accepted Herr K.'s sexual advance, but that there is, in the structure of hysteria as Lacan understands it, something barred at the level of desire which does not allow the female-hysteric to be the object cause (the "*a*") of man's desire. Dora, in Lacan's reading, does not wish to be a substitute for another woman, or an object of exchange, in the (phallic) sexual economy. But more than this, she must be kept at a safe distance from the other woman (as object) in order to desire. Dora's solution is to desire by privation and by proxy, through the other woman as object of the man's desire but at a safe remove. But the solution fails when the Real of the sexual advance shatters her fantasmatic positioning in the quadrille. Dora's desire, supported by the fantasy, collapses. "When desire collapses, the object becomes present, the object of the Other's demand, which indicates the certainty of jouissance" (Voruz 2007, 168). Desire, for Lacan, defends against jouissance because it introduces a gap. The gap is collapsed not only by the unwanted sexual advance but also by the pretense of nothingness as in, my wife gives me nothing.

Something is fundamentally ruptured not when Dora becomes an object of exchange but, as has already been said, when Herr K. says, *My wife means nothing to me*. For Lacan, Dora's unstated question was "If she is nothing to you, then what are you to me?" (2006h, 183). In his discussion of the case in *The Psychosis*, Lacan alters the question precipitating the almost instantaneous slap, "So, what can you be to me, then?" (1997, 91). The question of Dora's desire is front and central. Lacan says that Herr K. broke the spell Dora was under. But curiously, Lacan is nonchalant about the pregnancy fantasy to follow. "The latent pregnancy fantasy that followed this scene does not invalidate my interpretation, since it is well known that it occurs in hysterics precisely as a function of their identification with men" (2006h, 183).

Her homage to Frau K. is, in Lacan's reading, about the difficulty Dora has in accepting "herself as an object of desire…the problem of her condition is fundamentally that of accepting herself as a man's object of desire, and this is the mystery that motivates Dora' idolization of Frau K." (181). It is also what inspires Dora's fascination and study of the Madonna. Lacan suggests that Dora becomes a worshipper not of other, older, maternal-women as objects so much as she is looking, in these object-images and figures for a Christian solution to the impasse "by making women the object of a divine desire or a transcendent object of desire, which amounts to the same thing" (181).

Both Lacan and Ettinger know that Dora is raptured by Frau K and not Herr K. as Freud initially thought. Lacan refers to Dora's "fascinated attachment to Frau K ("her adorable white body")" along with the way she and Frau K are "mutual ambassadors of their desires regarding Dora's father" (180). But we should not assume that Lacan, like Freud, makes Dora's father, or even Herr K., the central player in Dora's story. In his larger discussion of hysteria in "Psychoanalysis and Its Teaching," Lacan says that the "hysteric comes to know herself [*s'éprouve*] in the homage paid to another woman, and offers up the woman in whom she adores her own mystery to the man whose role she takes without being able to enjoy it [*en jouir*]" (2006i, 377–378).

What Lacan does not elaborate upon is the non-present centrality of the mother in the Dora case. He implies that there was frustration between Dora and her mother and comments on the way she is described in the case as orderly, cold, and unloving. But his main interest is not in the mother, the aunt, the K.'s governess (who Dora replaces), or even Frau K. (as subject). Rather, he is interested in how Dora turns to her father to give her the missing object (symbolically) that her mother denies her. But like the mother, the father has not got it (the missing object) due, in part, to his impotence, but also because the *Thing* (as object of desire) does not exist as such.

What I find interesting from an Ettingerian point of view, is that Lacan introduces what he calls another "plane" in the object relation whereby the gift (of the object) is something other than a lack. "Isn't there another dimension that is introduced into the object relation on the level where it is raised to the symbolic degree by the fact that the object may or may not be given?" (Lacan 2020, 131–132). This other dimension is not unlike the matrixial sub-stratum of concern to Ettinger. Moreover, when Lacan says that love is about making one of two, he is, in my view, articulating something akin to the non-visible trace like link (*a-link*) that Ettinger differentiates from *object a*. Lacan contends that it is not the object that is ever given but rather a "sign of love" (132). He stresses Dora's love for her father and its correlation with his diminution. "She loves him precisely for what he doesn't give her" (133). Part of what the case study of Dora illustrates for Lacan is how "there is no greater possible gift, no greater sign of love, than the gift of what one hasn't got" (132).

In the Lacanian reading, the problem is not that Herr K. makes an improper sexual advance toward Dora. The problem is that the something in the beyond which may be compared to the matrixial is reduced to nothing. This beyond is not dissimilar to the matrixial sub-stratum of concern to Ettinger. For Lacan, the beyond is where the woman, as wife, disappears from the symbolic circuit. Lacan, like Ettinger, knows that something vital to the Woman and to the m/Other is eclipsed by the Symbolic. What Herr K. means in the German *Ich habe nichts an meiner Frau* is that "there is nothing beyond his wife – *My wife is not included in the circuit*" (135).

Like Ettinger, Lacan knows that the wife and daughter are exchangeable objects in the kinship structures studied by Lévi-Strauss. Both Lacan and Ettinger also know that the way the Women is not integrated into the Symbolic system of exchange poses problems on the Feminine side. As discussed in previous chapters, Ettinger accuses Lacan of phallocentrism (a word that becomes a synonym for sexism), but they are both, albeit in different ways, trying to understand the functions and effects of the Feminine not-all inscribed in the Symbolic. Lacan reasons that Dora has to relinquish the paternal phallus as symbolic gift. If she does not, Dora "can conceive of nothing, subjectively speaking, that she might receive from others, that is to say, from another man" (136). She has, in other words, nothing of value to give. Lacan is not saying that women, like Dora, lack value as people, but that what there is to give, from the Feminine side, is lacking. This is not a commentary on the value of the Feminine, but on the way elements of the Feminine do not get registered on the Symbolic plain.

In Lacan's account, hysterics, like Dora, struggle to situate themselves symbolically. "Dora knows neither where to locate herself, nor where she is, nor what she is meant for, nor what love is meant for" (138). Her interest in love takes the form of a symptomatic question, of what it means to be a woman. For Lacan, Dora does not become a woman. What Dora, like the case of the homosexual woman also analyzed by Freud demonstrates, in Lacan's reading, is "how one can love someone not only for what that person has, but literally for what the person doesn't have, for the symbolic penis she knows she will not find in the lady" (137).

While the Lacanian interpretation of hysteria is very different from the Ettingerian reading of hysteria, it is noteworthy that for Lacan the hysteric is, to some degree, like the Ettingerian Woman insofar as the hysteric is not an undivided subject. The hysteric speaks to the master from her positioning as a divided subject and, in so doing, mines unconscious content subject to repression. In "The Function and Field of Speech and Language in Psychoanalysis," Lacan writes that "the ambiguity of [the] hysterical revelation is…that it presents us with the *birth* of true speech, and thereby brings us up against the reality of what is neither true nor false" (2006l, 212, emphasis added).

In other words, the hysteric will not submit to the master's discourse predicated upon the primordial signifier. Her bodily symptoms indicate, among other things, that there is an otherness relevant to her being unbound by the signifier. As summarized by Voruz, the "master acquires mastery over his body through the signifier; the hysteric refuses this one-ifying power of the master-signifier" (2007, 176). If the hysteric exists with and alongside an Other she is not altogether different from the Ettingerian subject for whom not-sharing with the Other (as *non-I*) is an option. The hysteric, like the Feminine not-all, exists, at least in part, beyond the phallic premise (of the one). Another way to make the point is to say that both the Ettingerian woman and the Lacanian hysteric exist in a state of Symbolic exception.

In Lacanian terms, the Ettingerian Woman and the hysteric may be said to articulate the Feminine state of exception in terms of the not-all. There are, for Lacan, three positions a woman can occupy: she can "be" the phallus (what a man lacks); she can be the object cause of his desire (*objet a*); or she condescends to being the man's symptom upon which his *jouissance* is fixated (Soler 2002, 102). The hysteric refuses these three options. Moreover, the hysteric underscores the inability of the phallic signifier to make a sexual difference, a sexual relation (at least, from the phallic angle).

Conclusion

In my interpretation, Lacan does not sideline questions relating to the Feminine in the Dora case. In fact, Lacan foregrounds the significance of Dora's desire and faults Freud for not recognizing the significance of the Madonna (as maternal stand-in). Lacan insists that Freud's error in interpreting the case has to do with his inability to understand that Dora's willingness to be an accomplice in her father's affair was to preserve her own relation to her father's mistress.

What is even more interesting, from an Ettingerian perspective, is the way Lacan says that there is "something that belongs to *another realm*, yet which also carries considerable weight, [that] is playing a constant role in Dora's libidinal bond with Frau K." (2020, 130, emphasis added). Lacan does not elaborate upon his reference to "another realm" but it sounds strikingly similar to Ettinger's matrixial sub-stratum. He also, two paragraphs later, mentions the word matrix (*Urbild* in German) as that which is a narcissistic founding of the ego involving the "constitution of this imaginary function known as the ego" (Lacan 2020, 130–131). Although there is no ego or narcissism in the Ettingerian subject, Lacan's writing on the subject-to-subject relationship calls to mind the Ettingerian subject as several (severality). In his discussion of the transference as related to Dora, Lacan says:

> What must be understood about psychoanalytic experience is that it proceeds entirely in this subject-to-subject relationship, which means that it preserves a dimension that is irreducible to any psychology considered to be the objectification of certain of an individual's properties" (2006h, 176).

What Lacan refers to as a subject-to-subject relationship coincides with the Ettingerian notion of the subject-as-encounter. But where Lacan places emphasis upon language in subjectification, Ettinger is interested in non-verbal transmissions in the matrixial borderlinking.

Lacan also knows, like Freud, that illnesses speak and that these illnesses take on a particular significance for hysterics. His explanation for not privileging the "non-verbal aspects of behavior in the psychological maneuver" (2006h, 177) is that it reduces the analysand, in this case

Dora, to an object (as she became for Freud). Lacan uses the Dora case and, more specifically, the way Freud failed to uphold the psychoanalytic mandate to prioritize dialectical questions relating to desire, to illustrate the dangers of *homo psychologicus*. While Lacan does not define *homo psychologicus* in this presentation, it refers to a rational psychological calculous leading to the prioritizing not only observable behaviors, but desires that can be elicited and known and made transparent without contradiction or nuance. Freud's certainty that Dora desired Herr K., coupled with the way he, in Lacan's critique, stopped asking enigmatic questions about her desire, was a problem not only because it, in effect, thwarted and ended the analysis, but because it is un-psychoanalytic.

Lacan says that Dora leaves Freud with a "Mona Lisa smile" (183). There is something enigmatic in the half-smile painted by Da Vinci that Lacan likens to Dora's desire. There is, as Lacan knows, something more to the story that Dora does not say, and that Freud misses in his preoccupation with the adult male figures in the case. If we are going to come closer to the truth (which Lacan famously says can only be half-said), a dialectical approach to Dora's desire is, for Lacan, necessary. Freud should not have fixated upon what or who Dora desires. He should have first asked "who desires in Dora" (Lacan 1997, 174).

Ettinger may not disagree, but her focus is on the matrixial link (*a-link*) to the adult women in the Dora case. The *a-link* is, for Ettinger, unlike *object a* (non-object cause of desire) because it is not a cut. But let us be clear about the fact that the Lacanian cut is not only a severance, but a lure. In the discourse of the analyst, the "*a*" is in the position of agent. By remaining enigmatic and acting as a catalyst for desire (as opposed to being caught in the transference), Lacan says that analysts insert a lure. "What then does it mean to interpret transference? Nothing but to fill the emptiness of this standstill [in the analytic dialectic] with a lure. But even though it is deceptive, this lure serves a purpose by setting the whole process in motion anew" (Lacan 2006h, 184).

While Ettinger would not view the matrixial link in terms of the Lacanian non-object both would, in my summation, agree that there is something unseeable, relating to the Feminine, that functions like a tie in the interhuman, whether it be in the unconscious and in the transference for Lacan or in the matrixial borderlinking for Ettinger.

In the following chapter, I add a valuable Ettingerian supplement to the Lacanian lure by focusing on the significance of the m/Other in the *Ravishing of Lol Stein*.

Bibliography

Abraham, Nicolas, and Maria Torok. 1994. *The Shell and the Kernel: Renewals of Psychoanalysis, Volume 1*. Translated by Nicholas T. Rand. Vol. 1. University of Chicago Press. WorldCat.

Cavanagh, S. L. 2018. Transcryptums: An Ettingerian Reading of the Trans-subjective Landscape in Transparent" *Transgender Studies Quarterly, 6*(1): 20–42.

Duras, Marguerite. 1966. *The Ravishing of Lol Stein*. Translated by Richard Seaver. Grove Press.

Ettinger, Bracha. 2001. Matrixial Gaze and Screen: Other Than Phallic and Beyond the Late Lacan. In *Bodies of Resistance: New Phenomenologies of Politics, Agency, and Culture*, ed. Laura Doyle. Northwestern University Press.

Ettinger, Bracha L. 2006. Fascinance and the Girl-to-M/Other Matrixial Feminine Difference. In *Psychoanalysis and the Image*, ed. Griselda Pollock. Blackwell Publishing Ltd.

Ettinger, Bracha Lichtenberg. 2009. Fragilization and Resistance. *Studies in the Maternal* 1 (2): 1–31. https://doi.org/10.16995/sim.141.

Freud, Sigmund. 1963. *Dora: An Analysis of a Case of Hysteria*. 1997th ed. Simon and Schuster.

Gilman, Sander L., et al. 2022. *Hysteria beyond freud*. Univ of California Press.

Lacan, Jacques. 1997. *The Seminar of Jacques Lacan: The Psychoses 1955–1956, Book III*. Reprint edition. Translated by Jacques-Alain Miller and Russell Grigg. Norton.

Lacan, Jacques. 1998. *The Seminar of Jacques Lacan, Book XX: On Feminine Sexuality: The Limits of Love and Knowledge (Encore 1972–1973)*. Edited by Jacques-Alain Miller and Bruce Fink. WW Norton & Company.

Lacan, Jacques. 2006e. Guiding Remarks for a Conversation on Female Sexuality. In *Écrits: The First Complete Edition in English*. Translated by Bruce Fink. W.W. Norton & Company.

Lacan, Jacques. 2006h. Presentation on Transference. In *Écrits: The First Complete Edition in English*. Translated by Bruce Fink. W.W. Norton & Company.

Lacan, Jacques. 2006i. Psychoanalysis and Its Teaching. In *Écrits: The First Complete Edition in English*. Translated by Bruce Fink. W.W. Norton & Company.

Lacan, Jacques. 2006j. A Theoretical Introduction to the Functions of Psychoanalysis in Criminology. In *Écrits: The First Complete Edition in English*. Translated by Bruce Fink. W.W. Norton & Company.

Lacan, Jacques. 2006l. The Function and Field of Speech and Language in Psychoanalysis. In *Écrits: The First Complete Edition in English*. Translated by Bruce Fink. W.W. Norton & Company.

Lacan, Jacques. 2011. The Seminar of Jacques Lacan: Book X: Anxiety: 1962–1963. Unpublished manuscript. Translated by Cormac Gallagher.

Lacan, Jacques. 2020. *The Seminar. Book IV: The Object Relation (1956–57)*. Edited by Jacques-Alain Miller. Translated by AR Price. Polity Press.

Showalter, Elaine. 1985. *The Female Malady: Women, Madness, and English Culture*, 1830–1980. Penguin Books, New York.

Soler, Colette. 2002. What Does the Unconscious Know About Women. In *Reading Seminar XX: Lacan's Major Work on Love, Knowledge, and Feminine Sexuality*, SUNY Series in Psychoanalysis and Culture, ed. Suzanne Barnard and Bruce Fink. State University of New York Press.

Voruz, Véronique. 2007. A Lacanian Reading of Dora. In *The Later Lacan: An Introduction*, ed. Véronique Voruz and Bogdan Wolf. State University of New York Press.

6

Lol Stein: The Object, the Gaze, and the m/Other

Bracha L. Ettinger wrote about *The Ravishing of Lol Stein* in an article titled "Fascinance and the Girl-to-m/Other Matrixial Feminine Difference" (2006a). In this article, Ettinger uses the Freudian case study of Dora (discussed in the previous chapter) along with the character Lol Stein (Lola Valerie Stein) to elaborate upon the Other Sexual Difference (OSD). In *The Ravishing*, Duras (1966) portrays a woman, Lol Stein, troubled not by the way she is abandoned on the dance floor by her fiancé, who turns his attention to another woman, but by a need, ritually thwarted, to be included in a triadic scene of desire involving a maternal figure. Lol Stein watches, and waits, for the scene at the dance hall to repeat itself but in a way that involves her along with an-other woman so that she can, in Ettinger's interpretation, become a woman. Like what I think Lacan is getting at in his discussion of the passage-to-the-act (as related to the homosexual woman), Lol Stein, like Dora, want not only to leave a scene in which they are reduced to *object a* for the man, but also to move from the position of girl-daughter to woman. While Lacan reads the novel as animating what has been taken from us in love and how we

Portions of this chapter were previously published in: Cavanagh, Sheila L. (2025) "Jacques Lacan and the Ravishing of Lol Stein by Marguerite Duras." *Angelaki* 30.6: 52–69.

S. L. Cavanagh, *Bracha L. Ettinger and Jacques Lacan*, The Palgrave Lacan Series,
https://doi.org/10.1007/978-3-032-23293-9_6

must count ourselves three due, in part, to the presence of the Other in the missed romantic encounter, Ettinger introduces another axis of difference involving not only the m/Other, but the other woman, in the rapturous scene.

Through her interpretation of the novel, Ettinger develops key concepts relating to the matrixial including fascinance and the matrixial gaze as link-a. These concepts are offered as critical supplements to the Lacanian formulation of the gaze, the screen, and the image. Ettinger invites the reader to consider the role of the m/Other in the ravishing scene along with the other woman. What Lol Stein experiences is not best understood as arrested Oedipal development (in Freudian terms) or through the Lacanian formulation of *object a*, but, in Ettinger's assessment, through matrixial correlates relevant to the OSD involving the m/Other.

Like Ettinger, Lacan agrees that the gaze and the Other are central to the story. In his discussion of Lol Stein, Lacan stresses the significance of the fantasm and the way gaze of the Other orchestrates an "image of the self in which the other dresses you and in which you are dressed, and which, when you are robbed of it, lets you be just what underneath?" (Lacan 1987, 126). The absence of the dress unveils what Lol is left with, what has been "said about [her] that evening…what they said about you when you were a child, that you were never all there" (Lacan 124). Like Dora who was reduced to an object of exchange in her father's extramarital affair and the homosexual woman who is caught with her female lover by her father's proprietary gaze, Lol Stein is, on the dance floor, ensnared by the gaze Lacan calls a talisman that we are all eager to cast off (127).

In Ettinger's considered opinion, we must ask why and how the m/Other and the female friend are forgotten or, at least, sidelined in Lacan's discussion of the novel. In her estimate, Lol Stein does not suffer because she loses her fiancé or because she becomes identified with the loss in the gaze of the Other. Likewise, Dora does not (only) suffer because she has been, in Lacan's words, the object of an odious exchange—she for her Herr K.'s wife. Dora and Lol Stein are both made into objects (causes of desire for a man), but what hurts more profoundly is the absence, betrayal, or neglect of the mothers and their substitutes. Dora's mother was largely absent from her life and described as unavailable, depressed, and frail in

Freud's case study. Lol Stein's mother screams at the sight of the couple (Michael Richardson and Anne-Marie Stretter) on the dancefloor, a sight fascinating her daughter and when her mother dies Lol Stein does not shed a tear.

Ettinger does not dispute Lacan's reading of this classic text which appears on *Le Monde's 100 Books of the Century*. Nor does she challenge the formulation of the gaze that Lacan develops in *Seminar XI*. But she does introduce a matrixial supplement concerning the gaze and, in so doing, prioritizes female-to-female relations in the novel that Lacan ignores in his 1965 presentation.

In this chapter, I consider the omission of the m/Other in Lacan's homage to Duras, reinterpret the ravishing scene at Town Beach casino through an Ettingerian lens, and consider how Lol Stein's desire can be understood through the OSD. Like Dora, Lol Stein searches for an invents scenes containing, if not directly representing, a primordial encounter with the desire of the m/Other in the Ettingerian interpretation. Lol Stein and Dora were both animated by a primary sexual difference involving the m/Other and the other woman. Both need to repeat and re-stage a rapturous scene of desire because they are, with and alongside their own mothers, "rejected and out of place" (Ettinger 2006a, 74). The OSD is of great importance to the girl-becoming-woman in the Ettingerian frame because they are phantasmatically tied to the woman-beneath-the-m/Other in ways that differ for the boy-becoming-man (or woman).[1]

The m/Other

It is unfortunate that Lacan did not say something about the mother in his hommage to Marguerite Duras. Like Freud who fails to address the significance of the mother (along with the aunt) in the Dora case study, Lacan, interestingly, omits the question of the mother's desire at the ball

[1] As Ettinger explains, "Female subjects have double access to the matrixial sphere in the Real because they experience the womb both as an archaic out-site and past-side—out of chronological time as "anterior" (this is true for males as well)—and as an in-side and future-side—as an actual, future, and "posterior" time (whether they are mothers or not)" (2006d, 143).

in Town Beach where her scream precipitates her daughter's breakdown. But this does not stop him from asking questions about origin; where, for example, the author got the idea and inspiration for the character of Lol Stein. Calling to mind a toddler who mimics but does not understand speech, Lacan's first words to Duras were: "You don't know what you are saying!" (Rabaté 2019, 8). While he may have been condescending, belittling, and patronizing upon meeting the celebrated author in a bar at midnight, it is likely that he intended to underscore her brilliance in scripting an absence. Afterall, Duras illustrated what he calls *object a* (the mysterious thing causing desire) by, paradoxically, writing nothing about it. In his fascination with Duras and the character she creates in the novel, it is strange that he does not call upon the desire, discourse, and jouissance of the mother theorized in his own teachings.

This is an odd oversight given that all of Duras' writings bare the markings of her turbulent relationship with her mother. The author describes her mother in essays and interviews as a strict pedagogue, as unaffectionate, as having preferred her older brother to her, and as having become a father when her own biological father died (Duras 2019, 3). Her mother who "nearly went insane," who had "epileptic seizures that would rattle her until she lost consciousness" (Duras 2019, 4). Her mother who lost her life savings, who was duped into buying a worthless piece of land on which she could not grow anything (Duras 2019, 4). Duras explains that her mother's preference for her brother became "unbearable, especially when, egged on by him, she would beat me. She really roughed me up, yes, she would hurl herself at me when I slept around. She didn't slap me, she kicked me and hit me with a stick, with the help of my brother" (Duras 2019, 9).

Clarity did not come to Duras until later. Her relationship with her mother "came undone all at once" (Duras 2019, 8), likely when her first child was born or, as Duras speculates, when her film based on *The Sea Wall* (*Un barrage contre le Pacifique*) (1950) was made. *The Sea Wall* was partly autobiographical and shaped by Duras' impoverished adolescent life in French Indochina, the tragedy of the land purchase upon which not even rice could grow due to the dams ritually destroyed by the inundations of the China Sea (now the Pacific Ocean), and her mother's descent into madness. Referring to *The Sea Wall* (1967), Duras' mother told her daughter: "You should have waited for me to die" (Duras 2019, 8).

It could be argued that the subject of Durasian literature is not only shaped by the mother but also by the daughter's being in relation to the mother. Significantly, Lol Stein's father is only mentioned once in the book. He is a history professor from Germany who does not have an actual role in the novel. Her brother, nine years her senior, who lives in Paris is also not present. The other women and the m/other take on great significance in the novel. In fact, there were at least two mothers at the ball in Town Beach: Lol Stein's mother and Anne-Marie Stretter (who is both a mother and the ravishing other woman). The latter was described as tall and elegant in a way that Tatiana Karl (Lol Stein's childhood friend) said was upsetting. There are also two other women in the story who play a vital role in Lol Stein's life: Anne-Marie Stretter, who seduces her fiancé on the dancefloor, and Tatiana Karl who witnesses the traumatic scene and ten years later becomes Jacques Hold's lover.

Lol Stein says that "from the first moment that woman [Anne-Marie Stretter] walked into the room [the dance hall], I ceased to love my fiancé" (Duras 1966, 126). She is fascinated by the sight of Anne-Marie Stretter with Michael Richardson swaying on the dancefloor, and later by Tatiana Karl with Jacques Hold in the Forest Hotel of ill repute. Lol Stein waited on the sidelines of the dance floor at what Duras calls a tender age to be included in a rapturous scene that would have involved three, until her mother's harrowing scream. Lol Stein's mother, quite literally, pulls her daughter away from the rapturous scene that needed time to germinate. What is most tragic in the novel from an Ettingerian standpoint is the way the "premature evacuation [from the scene of desire transpiring on the dance floor] creates an unconscious move in which the subject is repetitively rejected: a repetitive phantasmatic scene of rejection from a matrixial femininity" (Ettinger 2006a, 69).

There is something not only about the couple, but about the desire and desirability of the Other woman that Lol Stein longs to see and partake in. Lol Stein's fantasies are not phallic (anchored to *object a*). Nor are they lesbian or even heterosexual but, rather, matrixial (including others as *non-I's*). In the novel, Jacques Hold is both narrator and character. He knows that he is not the object of attraction but the vector through which

Lol Stein searches for something, *but what?* He is cast in a ravishing scene designed by Lol Stein, not unlike a psychoanalyst positioned in the fantasy of an analysand. Jacques Hold says, "No one loves Tatiana in me. I belong to a perspective which she [Lol Stein] is in the process of constructing with impressive obstinacy…Tatiana, little by little, is forcing her way in, is breaking down the doors" (Duras 1966, 122). The novel is about the coming together of the two women, not romantically (or sexually), but, in Ettingerian terms, as partners in difference. Jacques Hold discovers that Tatiana Karl "has eyes only for Lol" and that he exists for her in an "oblique angle to Tatiana [Karl]" (137). Toward the end of the novel, Jacques Hold knows that he exists with and between the two women and says that he "had them both [Tatiana Karl and Lol Stein], enclosed within me" (156) which could be read in two ways: as him possessing both women from a phallic angle; or as him being an aggregated subject (more than one) from a matrixial angle. We may conclude that Jacques Hold is *object a* for both women in Lacanian terms, but for Ettinger, he is a part of the matrixial web (or plait of several[2]), even if the woman in him referred to as the "Tatiana in me" goes unloved.[3]

Read from an Ettingerian perspective, Jacques Hold not only narrates the matrixial primal scene for the reader but is, himself, part of it. Jacques Hold becomes part of a "future which she [Lol Stein] alone controls without knowing it" (121). He is not the object desired but a pawn in Lol Stein's fantasy. But Jacques Hold who, interestingly, shares the same given name as Jacques Lacan is also a pseudo-analyst. The reader depends upon his narrative interpretation to follow the plot. It may be that Jacques Hold is, like Jacques Lacan, interested in the Woman who does not exist. When Tatiana Karl undresses for Jacques Hold, he sees the woman he does not love, but focuses on the hollows of her body, where her "skin is thin…[and] white" (123), translucent. He searches for the void in Tatiana Karl where Lol Stein might be. Tatiana Karl surrenders to Jacques Hold.

---

[2] Much like Lacan's discussion of the *sinthôme* in his later work, Ettinger regards the matrixial plait-of-several as strong enough to stave off psychosis when the becoming-subject is ejected from a formative encounter-event.

[3] Jacques Hold knows that when Tatiana Karl asks him how he knows "such things about Lol" (Duras 1966, 140), she is really asking "how do you know such things when a woman doesn't? another woman who could be Lol Stein" (Duras 1966, 140).

She "knows how to let herself go" (124) as he turns her every which way in their love making. Afterward, Tatiana Karl says "with her head hidden beneath the sheet, she's not me, is she?" (125). Both Tatiana Karl and Lol Stein are not there fully for Jacques Hold. But viewed through an Ettingerian lens, both women are there: they are borderlinked in a Feminine transitive relation that Hold cannot describe or interpret in full.

The triangle Duras devises in the plot captures both phallic jouissance, as theorized by Lacan, and the Other (Feminine) jouissance relevant, as I suggest, to the Ettingerian borderlinking. For Lacan, the tragedy Duras depicts is inevitable. We are all alienated by the signifier and cut by lack which freezes us in the time and place of the Other's gaze. The sexual relation Lol Stein might have had—be it with Michael Richardson, John Bedford (Lol Stein's non-descript husband) or, later, with Jacques Hold—was always, from the Lacanian start, impossible. Ettinger's intervention is to suggest that Lol Stein's desire was not about the phallic object (the man or *object a*), but about the OSD and the other woman with whom she can and does relate.

As Duras writes in the novel, Lol Stein "loves the man who must love Tatiana" (122). As with Frau K. in the case study of Dora, the Other woman cannot be forgotten. Like all subjects, Lol Stein is inhabited by the Lacanian Other, the Other who occupies and speaks in me. But for Ettinger this inhabitation does not involve an absolute Other. When Jacques Hold stares at and ogles other women, Lol Stein gives "a start, as though he had done it to her" (44). What Ettinger calls the Feminine transitive relation is written into the plot. Consider also that there is something more than tenderness in Lol Stein's refusal to let Jacques Hold leave Tatiana Karl; even when the sex he has with Tatiana Karl is staged for Lol Stein's voyeuristic eyes. After having twice watched Jack Hold make love to Tatiana Karl from the rye field, Lol Stein says: "When you look at Tatiana the way you did the other evening, without seeing her, I have the feeling I'm remembering someone I'd forgotten" (165).

Is she remembering who she was before the ball? Or is Lol Stein seeing Tatiana Karl at the ball, the friend who remained by her side the entire night? Maybe she remembers that she, Lol Stein, is not there, at least not in full as others said. In Lacanian terms, she may be recalling a void or loss where the *object a* comes to be, but in Ettingerian terms, it is more likely that she recalls a ravishing matrixial scene analogous to what precedes Dora's breakdown; a scene involving the matrixial Feminine and the m/Other occluded in the Lacanian corpus.

The Ravishing Matrixial Scene

While Lacan writes about jouissance (a painful pleasure) and repetition, Ettinger writes about ravishing, as in the ravishing of Lol Stein. There is jouissance in ravishing, but from a matrixial perspective, it is tranformative. Ravishing is not about the way we are subject to the gaze of the Other (as *object a*) or about the way the Woman does not exist in the Symbolic. Nor is it about a lack in being or a painful repetition whereby a subject, like Lol Stein, experiences a masochistic or self-effacing jouissance. Ettinger contends that the ravishing is about an intensification felt on the precipice of a metramorphic change in and between partial-subjects in a shared matrixial web. Lol Stein, like Dora, longed for a change in the borderlinking to enable a passage into the position of woman. In the Ettingerian analysis, both Lol Stein and Dora are waiting, almost ritually, for the "blinding, puzzling, and slippery [matrixial] *encounter*" (2006a, 69) with an other-woman-m/Other. The wish is to be included in a rapturous encounter, to see, be seen, and to partake in it through to completion, so that the girl-daughters may become, by proxy, women in a shared matrixial borderspace. But for both Dora and Lol Stein, something was interrupted in the image, in the way they looked and waited, leaving them suspended in time, unable to complete the transition. Much like Dora stared at the Madonna, "Lol looked and looked, but she was torn away from the image too soon. An instance of differentiation on the long path of transformation from girlhood to womanhood was arrested" (62).

What Lol Stein needs is, for Ettinger, not unlike what Dora needs. They are not needing to be desired by men (or phallic subjects), but to know that the m/Other-Woman is desired by the lover and that she remain on the scene.

> For the Girl, the Lover must be unable to live without an m/Other-Woman; her coming into being depends on this. The coming-into-being in woman-

> hood of the Girl depends on the unconditional ravishing of the m/Other-Woman as such, and on her own both inclusion and exclusion from a scene that will give birth to her differentiated woman-self. (86)

In my reading, Ettinger is not ascribing to a classical romance genre whereby the woman-heroine is all or, in Lacanian terms, phallic. Rather, she is underscoring the primary importance of the m/Other-Woman to the girl-daughter-becoming-woman. While writing on the mother–daughter relation in psychoanalysis often positions the mother and daughter in competition for the husband-father's affections, Ettinger contends that the girl-daughter needs the m/Other or Other woman to be not only desired, but preferred. She writes that the girl-becoming-woman needs the lover (whomever they may be) to "prefer the m/Other-beneath-the-woman to the Woman-beneath-the-Girl" (86).

In Ettingerian terms, the ravishing is a binding in difference as opposed to a severance or psychotic disintegration. Although Lol Stein is not psychotic or a hysteric in Ettinger's analysis, she animates, for Ettinger, the dangers, or psychic fatalities, precipitated by a situation whereby the girl-becoming-woman cannot locate herself phantasmatically in a ravishing scene of desire involving the m/Other. While Lacan does not propose that Lol Stein is fused with the m/Other or that the daughter-mother relation is psychotic, there is, in Ettinger's reading, a way that Lacanian theory does not leave room to consider the subjectivizing potential of the borderlinking with-in, to and beside the m/Other. For Lacan, the child-subject needs the father (as paternal mediator) to interdict the desire of the m/Other. When there is no lack (or triangulation), the mother's desire and demand produces anguish (*angoisse*) in the child-subject. I will return to Lacan's writing on the m/Other in the conclusion, but suffice here to say that for Ettinger, Lacan regards what she calls the Feminine-matrixial borderlinking as, potentially, psychotic and predicated upon fusion. She states: "Unlike Lacan, I propose that we see in the mother-child common 'cloth' transgression and not fusion, braiding and not melting" (78).

In Ettinger's analysis of Lol Stein and her abrupt ejection from the ravaging scene on the dance floor that would have enabled her to complete a pass from girl-to-woman, Ettinger writes:

> A ravishing m/Other-Event-Encounter appears in front of the subject who is, herself, co-emerging with her and is in the process of becoming a woman, as if *it* is materialized in reality by an encounter between a woman and an-other (the Lover, a man in these cases, but who is not necessarily a male subject in my view) – an encounter in which the subject could have found a site for herself in order to continue this process in a satisfactory manner, but out of which *the subject is prematurely evacuated.* (68)

What must be understood in the Ettingerian analytic is the way becoming is not individual but occurs with-in encounters with others and that the m/Other (or substitute) is, for the girl-becoming-woman, of singular importance. Ettinger describes Lol Stein's premature evacuation from the phantasmatic scene as a subjective exile, an aborted encounter in the matrixial.

Ettinger would, no doubt, agree with the character Tatiana Karl who traces Lol Stein's "illness" (Duras 1966, 2) back before the night of the dance at Town Beach casino: "there was already something lacking in Lol, something which kept her from being, in Tatiana Karl's words, 'there'" (3). The ball was not the main event but, rather, the occasion for remembering something relevant to the m/Other that escapes consciousness. Ettinger likens the ravishing scene at Town Beach to an echo of the primal scene of birth. Much like the infant emerges from the mother, Lol Stein waits for, and repeats, a scene whereby she may be reborn as a woman in fascinance. The ravishing matrixial scene in Ettingerian theory is shocking because it does not bar the woman-m/Other and is Real (outside language). "It is an unbelievable, unexpected scene of passion, that is traumatic and traumatizing, and that produces a stupefied becoming-subject outside language, in front of the non-gaze of a woman-mother in relationship with her own lover" (Ettinger 2006a, 77).

The sexual difference of concern to Ettinger is impossible because, as lovers, we relate to *object a* as distinct from our partners, Ettinger contends that a sexual relation is possible in the matrixial due, in part, to the *a-link*. But let us consider that the *object a* and the *a-link* may have more in common than Ettinger presumes. Lacan explains that the *Thing* (or *das*

Ding) is the "most archaic of objects" (Lacan, Jacques 1992, 106) to which the subject is attached. In fact, Lacan defines *das Ding* as the "beyond-of-the-signified" (1992, 54) and as the "excluded interior" (1992, 101). He links the beyond of the signified to the mother and to her desire. Likewise, the sexual difference of concern to involves the m/Other, but she prioritizes the girl-becoming-woman's borderlinking to the m/Other. Sexual relations in the matrixial co-occur along shared but differentiated strings. They are presented as non-Oedipal and thus not phallic. For Ettinger, the OSD is about a "dawning and vanishing link with the m/Other who is a subjectivizing transformative agency in her position of a subject-in-resonance-with and in co-affection with the I" (Ettinger 2006a, 71). I will return to the question of the dawning and vanishing link in the next chapter on Antigone and consider its relation to the radiant splendor of Antigone as Lacan puts it. But for now, suffice to say that Ettinger focuses on the rapturous scene where the girl-becoming-woman needs the m/Other to desire and to be desired.

What fascinates Lol Stein is a compassionate and erotic borderlinking to the woman-Other-mother that Ettinger explicates in terms of fascinance. Fascinance involves desire and adoration but not in Oedipal terms. It is subjectivizing and ravishing (74), phantasmatic and Real. The matrixial primal scene is a rapturous encounter-event where change and transformation co-occur in and between partial subjects in the trans-subjective dimension.

The primal matrixial scene cannot be seen although it can be felt and apprehended in a matrixial web or plait of several. Ettinger describes the matrixial gaze as an affective swerve involving multiple others in a shared copoietic[4] web. It is not intersubjective, but trans-subjective and involves many partial-subjects as distinct from individual subjects. Ettinger describes a trans-subjective matrixial alliance whereby desire and jouissance is in and of the borderlinking in a metramorphic scene of change and transgression. This is to say that what is rapturous is not a jouissance of the object (as cause of desire), but a jouissance of co-emergence. The

[4] Copoietics involve transformational potentiality and is closely linked to metramorphosis. It takes place along "aesthetic and ethical unconscious paths: strings and threads, and produces a particular kind of knowledge" (Ettinger 2005, 703).

co-emergence "enables both an assembling and an exchange of psychic imprints, psychic transformation, and a process of growing differentiation in the course of further distinction and separation-in-proximity" (71). The OSD is not about the sexual non-relation as Lacan describes it in his seminar on feminine sexuality, but about differentiation and change in resonance and co-affectation.

Feminine Incest and Matrixial Time

In his essay "Guiding Remarks for a Convention on Female Sexuality," Lacan highlights the analytic myth relating to incest. He asks, "Why does the analytic myth come up short concerning the prohibition of incest between father and daughter" (Lacan 2006e, 619). Ettinger might agree that sexual prohibitions governing the girl child and mother relation are stronger than those prohibiting the girl child and father relation (and statistics relating to incest and child sexual abuse bare this out). But she approaches the question from another angle. By focusing on the life-generating imperative of what she calls the incestuous scene of birth, Ettinger helps us to understand why, from a phallic angle, there is reluctance, if not a prohibition, upon theorizing pregnancy and the primal scene of birth in psychoanalysis.

What Ettinger calls "feminine incest" (2006a, 77) is foundational to human reproduction. Cultural prohibitions surrounding the mother and child, perhaps particularly the mother and the boy-son, index, for Ettinger, yet another way in which the narcissistic interests of the boy-son-becoming-man are prioritized over the interests of the girl-daughter-becoming-woman. Much like the way Freud thought it important for the boy-son to deny the womb and the mysteries of childbirth as discussed in Chap. 3, cultural prohibitions make it difficult to theorize the singular importance of the m/Other and her reproductive capacity. This is, for Ettinger, due, in part, to the reluctance to acknowledge Feminine incest. Feminine incest involves a "traumatic encounter in the Real whose paradigmatic matrix is the encounter inside the maternal womb appears and reveals to us that there is a basic human condition where transgression of borderlines is certain" (Ettinger 2006a, 78). The law of the phallus, as

Ettinger understands it, cannot prohibit, or preclude Feminine incest. This non-prohibited incest enabling birth is what gives texture and form to the OSD. Ettinger describes the Feminine incest essential to life as involving

> a primordial psychic field of transgressions between several participants who render and temporarily loosen their Oedipal borderlines, thus creating crossings between their traumas and jouissances, phantasms, and even desires, and enabling the trans-scripting of traces of the links in an assembly of the several (in "severality") outside of linear Oedipal time. (78)

Matrixial time is unlike Oedipal time and is not chronological. It is a time when the future traumatically meets the past. Lol Stein's fascination with Anne-Marie Stretter, the woman who is both a mother and who seems to hold the secret of desire, unfolds in matrixial time until it is interrupted and frozen in time. It is not the passing of time, but the way time seems to stop that led to Lol Stein's collapse. She needed more time than she had to metabolize the scene involving the blinding desirability of the "fatal-woman-Other-mother" (*femme-fatale-Autre-mère*) (68). The fatal-woman-Other-mother's desirability touches upon an unremembered Feminine incestuous scene. The fatal-woman-Other-mother is not an individual subject as such. Rather, she is the

> being of the ravishing m/Other-Thing-Event in-itself as becoming with-in encounter; this Woman-beneath-the-mother, always almost lost and longed-for and almost always not-yet found again, both outside (in reality) and inside the self (in phantasm), who shines through another woman who is relating to a man to whom the subject intimately relates as well. (68)

The matrixial scene at the Town Beach casino is turbulent and Real because it contains, but does not directly represent, something of the non-prohibited incest involving the m/Other. The OSD is enabled by the "impossibility of avoiding incestuous relations with the m/Other in the [late] phase of pregnancy" (76).[5]

[5] Matrixial incest (which is essential for life) must be distinguished from what Ettinger calls genital-phallic incest after-birth (which is traumatic).

Lol Stein was relating to the female m/other-woman figure until there was an interruption in the time of borderlinking. Lol Stein does not want the evening at the Town Beach casino to end; she needed more time to absorb something changing for all three characters in the border recesses of the image. As narrated by Jacques Hold, the "ball immured in its nocturnal light, would have contained all three of them, and they alone. Lol is positive of that: together they would have been saved from the advent of another day, of one more day at least" (Duras 1966, 38).

Lol Stein's gaze was interrupted by the light of day, and she became identified with a loss or lack that binds her to a missed encounter-event. In Ettingerian terms, Lol Stein's matrixial gaze was arrested: the times of the present, past, and future collapsed. With the first rays of morning dawn, Tatiana could see how Lol Stein, Michael Richardson, and Anne-Marie Stretter had aged; "all three of them had aged years and years, grown centuries older, that kind of age which lies lurking, within the insane" (9–10). Changes that could not be seen were felt acutely by all involved. These non-visible transformations "affected [everyone, including Michael Richardson]…Lol was watching…watching him change" (7). While his eyes grew brighter, there was "etched upon it [Michael Richardson's face], ancient, primordial pain" (7).

When Lol Stein returns to the casino with Jacques Hold a decade later, he tries to synchronize his look with hers. He recalls her memories. "I remembered events contiguous to those events she remembered having been present at, sharp profiles of similarities that vanished the moment they were seen into the dark night of the room" (170). Jacques Hold enters Lol Stein's primal scene. He sees Michael Richardson and Anne-Marie Sletter move toward her like a "slow moving comet, the primary maw of love, she still didn't realize what it meant" (170). He hears Lol Stein's mother scream. He takes in the dawn arriving. Lol Stein is looking again ten years later, this time with Jacques Hold. She is "seeing again what cannot be seen again" (171).

Fascinance

The vanishing spectacle is, for Ettinger, about fascinance. Lol Stein's desire is often described as enigmatic,[6] but for Ettinger, the character wants to be "co-re-born as a woman in relations of fascinance" (Ettinger 2006a, 85). Like Dora, Lol Stein did not have the experience of being caught in a desiring gaze by a maternal figure who would have enabled her to become a woman in relations of fascinance. As discussed in the previous chapter, "Fascinance is an aesthetic affect that operates in the prolongation and delaying of the time of encounter-event and allows a working-through of matrixial differentiating-in-jointness" (61). It is distinct from fascinum; a phallic gaze theorized by Lacan in *Seminar XI*. Fascinum arrests movement and kills life, much like the evil-eye. Fascinance is like a lingering gaze. There is, in the scene of fascinance, a prolongation of fantasy. It occurs when there is a wit(h)nessing of matrixial differentiating-in-jointness. It occurs with and in a "sensitive image, sound, touch, move, breath, etc." (Ettinger 2005, 703). Unlike the Lacanian formulation of the gaze as *fascinum*, which involves a freezing of the subject as spectacle, *fascinance* is the "transformational subjectivizing potentiality of a matrixial link (gaze or voice)" (Ettinger 2006a, 61).[7]

Matrixial fascinance involves Feminine figures (62) as distinct from females in biological terms, and thus includes men, like Jacques Hold, who tries to see what Lol Stein apprehends in the matrixial encounter-event. He sees that Lol Stein is, like Dora in Ettinger's analysis, fascinated by the Feminine. In both the fictive and real clinical case, the matrixial gaze was either arrested or held in abeyance which, from a matrixial perspective, is traumatizing. What interests Ettinger about Lol Stein and Dora is the way both experienced a breach in a moment that may have allowed them to become women. Something vital to the borderlinking with the female m/Other-woman figure was severed and they were cast

[6] In Namiko Haruki's (2012) Lacanian reading of the book, what Lol Stein wants is turned into the "very essence of a riddle" (Haruki) (*mot-trou*). Indeed, there is almost never a noun (or referent) following the verb phrase 'to want' as related to Lol Stein. Duras writes, for example, "She [Lol Stein] has wanted to for some time" (1966, 45).

[7] Ettinger's critique of fascinum is not only based on her reading of Lacan, but upon Barthes' writing on the photograph which deadens and arrests the subject in motion.

out of the ravishing "m/Other-Event-Encounter" (68, emphasis in original).

As noted in the previous chapter, Dora's mother was sickly (or perhaps depressed), her aunt dies, and her father's mistress betrays her. In Ettinger's reading, Dora is repeatedly disappointed, betrayed, and abandoned by the adult-women-mother figures in her life. She is set on a path of endless "wandering and repetitive exiles. It subjectivizes her as an orphan to the matrixial sphere, from now on and once again and perpetually" (69). Dora, like Lol Stein, could not complete the transition to woman and both were, consequently, left "eternally in a position of girls along the woman-to-woman differentiated string" (63). Like Lol Stein who is left in the matrixial lurch, Dora is, in her late teenage years, left in abeyance; in the position of girl-daughter without a maternal figure to enable a change in the borderlinking. "Even when she [Lol Stein] became a woman, a wife, and a mother, she remained a girl along the feminine-matrixial differentiated axis, unable to close the gap between these two poles: the girl's and the woman's" (63).

The gap between these two-poles is not only about what it means to become a woman and to insist upon the desire and desirability of the mother, but about the pain of occlusion in the Feminine dimension. How are we to understand the traumata of being a girl-about-to-become-a-woman when the mother, her substitutes (and semblants) are absent, indifferent to, or betray the girl occupying the position of daughter?

The Sinthôme

Ettinger's theorization of borderlinking in the matrixial weave gives us a way to understand the trauma of the girl-daughter in the maternal trans-subjective relation. Her writing on the matrixial weave calls to mind the Borromean knot of Lacan's later work. The Borromean knot functions to tie the three registers, the Symbolic, the Imaginary, and the Real, together when one (or more) registers do not link. Lacan introduces the *sinthôme* (an old word for symptom) in his later work (1975–1976) to account for the palliating effects of the symptom. The Lacanian *sinthôme* is jouissant and accomplished through a creative rendering of the symptom—thus, the symptom is not to be removed or excised, but to be subjectively employed and used to knot the Real to the Imaginary and the Symbolic. For Lacan, the other sex can be a *sinthôme* and while the "woman" is a *sinthôme* (symptom) of man she may also be a *sinthôme* for another woman. In both instances, the *sinthôme* is the other sex. As he explains, the sex to which one does not belong, which is to say a woman, is the *sinthôme* (2018).

Building upon Lacan's theorization of the *sinthôme*, Ettinger posits a uniquely Feminine *sinthôme*. While the Lacanian *sinthôme* functions to palliate the missing paternal metaphor (or Name of the Father), the Ettingerian *sinthôme* is relevant to the m/Other. Ettinger's formulation of the matrixial *sinthôme* is also used to interpret what she calls the Jocasta complex which I discuss in the following chapter on Antigone. Here, suffice to say that the Jocasta complex involves dilemmas and obstacles relevant to the girl-becoming-woman in the matrixial. Ettinger suggests that viewed from the perspective of the Feminine matrixial, the *sinthôme* may be seen as an "intersection that creates/invents/reveals/releases a potential desire from its dangerous …archaic zone" (2002, 225). It involves a swerve and a borderlinking "from/with-in and in contact with a Real 'touched' by the feminine *Thing*" (Ettinger 2004, 86). The Feminine *Thing* is like the Lacanian *Thing* (*das Ding*) as *object a*, but for Ettinger it links back to the m/Other and has a connecting as opposed to a cutting function.

The matrixial *sinthôme* engages a Feminine (non-phallic) sexual difference in Ettinger's view. She acknowledges that Lacan was, through his formulation of the *sinthôme* in his later years, signaling to the possibility of a Feminine rapport. For instance, he suggests that there may be something in the sexual non-rapport that works itself out from the perspective of the symptom. But Ettinger maintains that the matrixial *sinthôme*, unlike the Lacanian *sinthôme*, is a non-phallic sublimation (Ettinger 2001, 120). While questions remain about how the matrixial *sinthôme* differs from the Lacanian *sinthôme* when Lacan contends that the *sinthôme* is the Other sex (which is a woman), the Ettingerian *sinthôme* is described as involving a link to the m/Other. More specifically, the matrixial *sinthôme* is an erotic binding; a jouissance of the borderlinking.

This jouissant borderlinking, in my reading, calls to mind elements of the Other jouissance in Lacan's work. Lacan likens the Other jouissance to the experience of mystics and to women in general, who are animated by something that cannot be seen or said. The Other jouissance[8] may harken back to a void or lack or loss in being that Ettinger attributes the unremembered matrixial scene of birth. However we may theorize the Other jouissance, for both Ettinger and Lacan, there is a ravishing that they place on the Feminine side: a ravishing that is, for Ettinger, an Eros in the borderlinking and, for Lacan, a ravishing relating to the way elements of the Woman do not exist in the Symbolic.

Lacan's Other jouissance may be said to dissolve or decomplete the subject and is, like matrixial jouissance, fragilizing. But the fragilization is, for Ettinger, a subjectivizing borderlinking with the m/Other as opposed to a fading or disintegration. She explains that the trauma in co-emergence is about the process of "differentiating-in-jointness of the I with the archaic m/Other" (Ettinger 2006d, 124). This involves what Ettinger calls "*enjoy-sense (jouis-sens)*" (117). This enjoy-sense includes sensations, vibrations, pulsations, etc., of joint corpo-reality with-in-of the m/Other. It is a cause of desire but also fascination. In the ravishing matrixial encounter, Ettinger elucidates a trans-subjective matrixial alliance whereby desire and jouissance is in and of the borderlinking. The borderlinking involves a metramorphic scene of change, transformation, and transgression. This is to say that what is rapturous is not a jouissance of the object (as cause of desire), but a jouissance of co-emergence enabled by the *a-link* (or link a). The co-emergence "enables both an assembling and an exchange of psychic imprints, psychic transformation, and a process of growing differentiation in the course of further distinction and separation-in-proximity" (71).

[8] Jouissance contains what Lacan calls a "frightening core of the *destrudo*" (1992, 194).

The Wail of the Mother

Lol Stein is fascinated by Anne-Marie Stretter who is a mother and a ravishing other-woman. She arrives at the Ball with her daughter who is not even named let alone described in any detail by Duras. Without anyone knowing how, Anne-Marie Stretter seduces Michel Richardson, Lol Stein's fiancé. Lol Stein gazes in fascination until her own mother arrives at the ball unannounced and unexpected. Lol Stein's mother bursts onto the scene and tears her daughter away from a captivating image on the dance floor, the image of Michael Richardson and Anne-Marie Stretter dancing with eyes interlocked. A moment of differentiation along a matrixial string (as sinthomatic *a-link*) was severed. In Ettinger's words, "An instance of differentiation on the long path of transformation from girlhood to womanhood was arrested" (Ettinger 2006a, 62).

Let us remember that it was not when Anne-Marie Stretter captured the attention of her fiancé that Lol Stein broke down. By all accounts, Lol Stein seemed to enjoy watching the couple on the dance floor. She was not ravished by jealousy. Lol Stein seemed neither upset nor anxious, but fascinated. What froze the girl in a scene she repeats in different ways throughout the novel was precipitated by her mother's scream. The maternal intervention disabled what might have been an encounter with the other-woman in the mother represented by Anne-Marie Stretter. "Insulting and reviling them, she [Lol Stein's mother] asked them what they had done to her child" (Duras 1966, 11). No one seemed to know why or how her mother knew what had taken place on the dance floor, not having witnessed the clandestine exchange with her own maternal eyes. The wail of the mother sounded after finding her daughter camouflaged behind a cluster of green plants. Lol Stein felt her mother touch her as she lost her own grip on a nearby table.

> It was only then that she had realized, vaguely, that something was drawing to a close, without quite knowing what it might be. The screen which her mother formed between them and her was her first inkling of it. With a powerful shove of her hand, she knocked her mother down. The vague, emotional-filled wail ceased. (11–12)

As her mother's archaic moan grew silent Lol Stein began to scream. She did not want Michael Richardson or Anne-Marie Stretter to leave. She begged them to stay, screamed all sorts of things including a refrain subject to repetition throughout the novel: "It wasn't late, it was only the early summer dawn that made it seem later than it really was" (12). Lol Stein hurled herself up against the door in attempt to block the lovers' exit, but to no avail. They descended the stairs, one by one, and then when Lol Stein "could no longer see them, she slumped to the floor, unconscious" (12).

Lol Stein says, "Yes. I wasn't there any longer. They took me with them. When I woke up, they were gone…I don't understand who's there in my place" (127). Before the scene was brought to a premature end, Lol Stein was existing in the place of the other woman, Anne-Marie Stretter. Lol Stein was experiencing herself as a desired and desiring subject by proxy. Something transformative was happening and then everything stopped. She was partaking in the ravishing scene until something like a needle on a record player was lifted in a reckless manner, scratching a song-track Lol Stein was destined to repeat. Much like Dora responds to Herr K.'s sexual advance with a resounding slap by the lake, the sound of Lol Stein's mother shrieking brought everything to a halt.

Later in the novel, Lol Stein restages the scene, which Ettinger interprets in terms of fascinance, but this time involving Tatiana Karl (in place of Anne-Marie Stretter). With the help of Jacques Hold who does not resist her desire to recreate the evening at Town Beach, Lol Stein tries to become a woman. Ettinger describes Lol Stein as having been eternally caught in the position of girl-child. "She, therefore, remains an eternal child captured in a repetitive primal scene out of which she cannot emerge for lack of absorption in a gaze of fascinance. She was trapped by fascinance" (Ettinger 2006a, 66). As Ettinger explains in her discussion of the non-individual plait or shared psychic cloth (that is a matrixial reformulation of the Lacanian plait discussed in *Les non-dupes errant*), Lol does not become a woman which is, in Ettinger's paper on fascinance (2006a), anyone who "exhibits the intersections of knots or a multiplied plait, that is: a trans-individual fabric" (83).

In Lacanian terms we might say that Lol Stein was arrested by the gaze of the Other, frozen in the place and time of that formidable night. He is not wrong. But in Ettinger's account, fascinum is preceded by fascinance which requires a lingering, one might say, playful gaze. Had she not been torn from the image of her fiancé and Anne-Marie Sletter dancing so soon, so violently, Lol Stein may have been able to metabolize the change in the borderlinking. Ettinger explains that "Lol was bathing in *fascinance*, sharing the offering of a transforming fascinating-fascinated gaze, before it prematurely turned to fascinum" (Ettinger 2006a, 63). As Lacan explains in relation to the phallic gaze, fascinum mortifies the subject. "The anti-life, anti-movement function of this terminal point is the *fascinum*, and it is precisely one of the dimensions in which the power of the gaze is exercised directly" (Lacan 1998, 115). Ettinger does not seem to disagree. What happened to Lol Stein, in Ettingerian terms, is that the matrixial scene of fascinance occurring at the ball became an image, an image to which she is attached and bound to repeat.

Object a and the *a-Link*

Fascination in the matrixial scene is not unrelated to the Lacanian object cause of desire. *Object a* takes many forms in Lacan's teachings, but in his discussion of fascinum (1998) he refers to it as the "fascinatory element introduced by the gaze" (115). Seeing is subordinated to the gaze because the latter is moored by desire. Lacan notes, also, that we are fascinated by the *Thing* (*das Ding*) that seems to evacuate or gut us from the inside. Lol Stein is not only taken by the gaze of the Other but fascinated by it. She cannot separate from it. Lacan likens the *object a* to a "substance caught in the net of a shadow, and which, robbed of its shadow-swelling volume, holds out once again the tired lure of the shadow as if it were substance" (Lacan 2006g, 693). For Lol Stein, the evening of the ball, like the black dress and Tatiana's long black hair, are like the lure of the shadow in Lacan's exposition. The lure has the structure of an image's rim. Lacan describes the image as a "rim, an opening, a gap, where the constitution of the specular image shows its limit, [this] is the elective locus of anxiety" (2011, 108). Lacan further elaborates upon the rim as a frame, like a stage that conjures-up an edge. Like the edge of a mirror, the rim is a limit to what can be represented in the visual field.

The Lacanian formulation of *object a* is not, in my reading, incongruous with Ettinger's formulation of the *a-link*. But, in Ettinger's assessment, what Lacan calls *object a* has a borderline visibility (1996, 150) harkening back to primary relations with the m/Other. By this, she means that the derivatives of the lost maternal object has a presence in phantasy. "In the invisible screen of phantasy, the *objet a* is a non-specular object situated at the borderline of the subject's mirror images which are created by the Other" (150). This is to say that what lacks a signifier appears in the phantasy screen invisible to the naked eye. Ettinger is critical of how these non-visible appearances in the screen of phantasy are, in Lacanian theory, objectified in what she groups together and names "Woman-Other-Thing" (150). But regardless of what we call the missing objects conjured-up in and on the screen at the level of phantasy, they are, for Ettinger, access points to the OSD that cannot be delimited by what is given (in the mirror) to be seen.

For Ettinger, Lol Stein is fascinated by a matrixial scene that, while unseeable, is gleaned and felt from another angle, a scene that she returns to and repeats. Hence, the phantasmatic repetition structured by Lol Stein's desire. Lol Stein is waiting for something non-descript to be apprehended. This reading corresponds to Lacan's contention that something appears in the place of *object a*. For example, in Lacan's writing on anamorphosis, he considers how the intangible object causing desire has a non-optical visibility. An anamorphosis is a way of perceiving the object-Thing askance, in a partial or distorted form when, in a direct line of vision, it would be imperceptible. Lacan's anamorphosis is like an optical illusion that reveals something inside the subject outside the subject. It makes that which is invisible (the Real) not visible exactly, but apprehendable.

What is unique about the Ettingerian formulation of the matrixial gaze as a-link is that she highlights the affective and aesthetic dimensions of the anamorphosis and traces it back to the m/Other in more rigorous detail. The matrixial gaze[9] is not about optical illusions for Ettinger so

[9] The matrixial gaze is haptic, involving touching and co-mingling with the Other in the subject along with the Other's subjective presence. The touching gaze occurs in the "*beyond-the-phallus* dimension" (2006d, 42).

much as it is about a touching, haptic gaze that is binding, as opposed to cutting, splitting or castrating. The matrixial gaze is a point of contact that recalls the m/Other and, as Ettinger concedes, the phallic gaze of Lacan's teachings is also not entirely phallic. Indeed, her formulation of the matrixial gaze is developed in relation to the Lacanian gaze. The matrixial gaze, which is a matrixial supplement to the phallic gaze, "indicates that relations are possible between a subject and another subject who looks at him/her without being observed" (Ettinger 2006d, 55). Ettinger explains that the "phallic gaze alleges that something was there and is now lost. The matrixial gaze indicates that something happened and the event has passed, and also that someones were there and these someones have already changed" (119). This "someone" who is, first and foremost, the m/Other is, ultimately, sublimated but, nevertheless, felt beyond the visible.

Lol Stein felt something as she stared at Anne-Marie Stretter on the dancefloor with her fiancé that could not be said or seen. Whatever this something was, it is described by Ettinger as involving the secrets and essence of femininity. There *was* something different about Anne-Marie Stretter that others at the ball studied closely. "What had she, Anne-Marie Stretter, experienced that other women had missed?" (Duras 1966, 6). This woman who carried herself with a "self-assured boldness" (6). The poise and beauty of Anne-Marie Stretter was not of the conventional sort. She arrived not at the ball exactly, but in Lol Stein's eyes, "at what appeared to be a gay, a dazzling pessimism, a smiling indolence as light as a hint, as ashes" (6). The self-possession of Anne-Marie Stretter resembles the beauty and blinding splendor of Antigone who adheres to a Feminine law at odds with the patriarchal law of her uncle, the King of Thebes (to be discussed in the next chapter). People at the Town Beach ball speculated about how Anne-Marie Stretter caught Richardson's attention. How did her gaze command his attention? *Had she surreptitiously looked at him*? "*Had this non-look of hers swept over him as it took in the ballroom*" (6)?

What does Lol Stein see?

What Lol Stein cannot see at Town Beach overtakes the ball on that formidable night and captivates everyone in attendance. For Ettinger, matrixial affects saturate the dancehall and are transmitted by a matrixial gaze. If Lol Stein's vacant look is not enough to animate the Feminine dimension that cannot be written, at least not exactly, in the novel, Duras gives us a second and more concrete example. Anne-Marie Stretter is described as having a visual impairment: "her gaze—from close-up one could see that this defect stemmed from an almost painful discoloration of the pupil—was diffused over the entire surface of her eyes, and was hard to meet" (Duras 1966, 6). Like Lacan's stain that dominates the screen of fantasy, Lol Stein searches and waits for something to appear beyond the visual field.

For Lacan, the gaze is a kind of trace appearing in the screen of a subject's phantasy. It is formed prior to the eye's capacity to see. We do not appear in the gaze as ourselves, but only as a stain in the screen that we may liken to an effacement. As Ettinger explains, in the Lacanian gaze "we do not appear to ourselves – except as a *stain* in the picture, or as a screen between the gaze and the picture, or as a stain on the screen" (Ettinger 2006d, 98). The gaze functions in the orbit of the Other, whereas the eye looks from the position of the subject. There is a radical discord between the gaze and the eye, and the image. Like the matrixial *a-link*, *object a* cannot be generated as an image. But the matrixial *object a* (or *a-link*) does have, as Ettinger explains, a borderline visibility. The *a-link* is "before subjective time: an ever too-early, forever too-late time-and-place…between conception and birth" (130–31).

The vanishing matrixial link Lol Stein cannot see is often mistaken for a masochistic or melancholic investment in an impossible loss (Haruki 2012). From an Ettingerian perspective, Lol Stein is not looking for proof of origins or a return to the primal scene of conception. She needs to apprehend something non-visual crucial to her being in the matrixial. As Duras writes in the novel (through the character/narrator Jacques Hold), "She, who does not see herself, is thus seen, in others. Therein lies the omnipotence of this substance whereof she [Lol Stein] is made, without any particular ties" (Duras 1966, 45). Perhaps, it is the matrixial sinthomatic tie that Lol Stein longs to enable, a tie that involves Anne-marie Stretter. "Replaced by that woman…Lol holds her breath as this woman's body appears to this man, her own fades, fades, voluptuous pleasure, from the world" (40). But the journey is incomplete. What Duras describes to us as the "divesting of Anne-Marie Stretter's dress…this velvet annihilation of her own person…[was not brought] to its conclusion" (40).

The novel is structured by the scene Lol Stein repeats in which she is stripped (*dérobée*) of her lover, but not because she wants the man who she is said to have lost. When Jacques Hold (a stand-in for Michael Richardson) professes his love to Lol Stein the character will not allow him to break-up with Tatiana Karl. In fact, Lol Stein breaks down when she spends the night with Jacques Hold at the Town Beach dance hall without her schoolgirl friend. Lol Stein needs to see Michael Richardson desiring Anne-Marie Stretter, like she needs to see Jacques Hold desiring Tatiana Karl. It is as if these women come into existence not through the men exactly, but through the gaze of the Other woman waiting and watching on the side-lines.

Tatiana Karl is the other woman who watches Lol Stein from an oblique angle. She is there when Lol Stein collapses on the sidelines of the dance floor. She is there with Jacques Hold when Lol Stein watches their lovemaking from the rye field. She was, before any of the men in the novel, the first to dance (in her childhood days), with Lol Stein. Tatiana Karl also knows that something vital to Lol Stein's being had been lost, even before the Ball at Town Beach. She knows this better than does Jacques Hold who most closely resembles the psychoanalyst in the novel. Tatiana Karl does not worry about her friend's sanity; she but worries that her friend may have lost her madness.[10] Tatiana Karl is not concerned about curing Lol Stein's so-called condition, or with the residual symptoms of her breakdown so much as she is concerned about whether Lol Stein has lost something resonate with a Feminine Eros: "One should

[10] We should question whether Lol Stein is, indeed, mad. She is described by Duras as apathetic, uninvested in life, bored, without direction and feeling. Lol Stein loses something central to her being without losing functionality. What interests Ettinger is the way Lol Stein is distracted by an apparition, the image of something relevant to the Feminine that cannot be seen by the naked eye.

never be completely cured of one's passion" (67) as written in the text. The character, Tatiana Karl, is skeptical of the cure and knows that the symptom is integral to Lol Stein's being as a desiring subject.

When Jacques Hold finally makes love to Lol Stein at the end of the novel, she loses herself again in something akin to madness—like she did at the Town Beach casino. But this time she does so while establishing a borderlinking to Tatiana Karl; thus, making a fantasmatic trouple (or plait of three) with Jacques Hold in the place of the knot (Lacan) or borderlinking (Ettinger).[11]

As Lacan would agree, there is always an Other in love complicating the couple and Lol Stein gives the Other a Feminine name. Lol Stein does not take the surname Hold as one might expect in a marriage following love-making in the late post-war period, but adds her friend's name to her own name by addressing herself as "Tatiana Karl and Lol Stein" (179). She exists with and alongside the other woman (Tatiana Karl). In Ettingerian terms, the combined feminine names signify a transitive Feminine relation. This is not a regressive transitivism so much as it is an expression of a matrixial triangle involving the Other woman. Although there are differences in each theorization, both Ettinger and Lacan seem to agree that the Other (woman) is there and that the m/Other is foundational to the structure of desire in the *sinthômatic* knot (Lacan) and Feminine borderlinking (Ettinger).

While Lacan may be faulted for neglecting the m/Other in his presentation on the Duras novel, he, like Ettinger, notices the central importance of the triangle. Lacan reads *The Ravishing* as animating what has been taken from us in love and how we must count ourselves three due, in part, to the presence of the Other in the missed romantic encounter. Specifically, he says there is a "threefold being, in which Lol is suspended" (Lacan 1987 [1966], 127). His interest in the three is not, in my

[11] Duras composes what Ettinger calls a "triple cross-subjectivity" (2006a, 76). This cross-subjectivity is not to be understood on the intersubjective plain but, rather, on the terrain of the sub-Symbolic where we are all partial-subjects (more than one). In her discussion of Lol Stein in the Marguerite Dura novel, Ettinger explains that "The transgression of subjective borderlines between the individuals creates momentarily not a single separated subject (a Girl) vis-à-vis another subject (a Woman, a Mother) or even a third subject (a Man), but an aggregated subjectivity or what I call *subjectivity-of-the-several in encounter-event* that, in a blissful Real or in a traumatic and phantasmatic way, opens a path for cross-inscription" (Ettinger 2006a, 73).

assessment, about a wish to undermine the significance of each individual subject in the triangles Duras depicts, much less the mother. Rather, he intends to stress the way the m/other is present in the braid of three, even when she cannot be named as such.[12]

In the following chapter on Antigone, I explore what Ettinger refers to as a transgression-with-in-to-the-Feminine of relevance to the Jocasta complex. In so doing, I consider whether Lacan, in his reading of the play, forgets or, rather, cannot name the m/Other in his commentary on psychoanalytic ethics because she is, in his view, a condition of speech.

Bibliography

Duras, Marguerite. 1966. *The Ravishing of Lol Stein*. Translated by Richard Seaver. Grove Press.

Duras, Marguerite. 2019. Motherhood Makes You Obscene. *The Paris Review*, October 1. https://www.theparisreview.org/blog/2019/10/01/motherhood-makes-you-obscene/.

Ettinger, Bracha. 1996. Metramorphic Borderlinks and Matrixial Borderspace. In *Rethinking Borders*, ed. John C. Welchman. University of Minnesota Press.

Ettinger, Bracha. 2001. Matrixial Gaze and Screen: Other Than Phallic and Beyond the Late Lacan. In *Bodies of Resistance: New Phenomenologies of Politics, Agency, and Culture*, ed. Laura Doyle. Northwestern University Press.

Ettinger, Bracha Lichtenberg. 2002. Trans-Subjective Transferential Borderspace. In *A Shock to Thought: Expression after Deleuze and Guattari*. Routledge.

Ettinger, Bracha. 2004. Weaving a Woman Artist With-in the Matrixial Encounter-Event. *Theory, Culture & Society* 21 (1): 69–94.

Ettinger, Bracha. 2005. Copoiesis. *Ephemera: Theory & Politics in Organization* 5 (X): 703–713.

[12] Lacan explains that the mother exists within the realm of prohibited objects and cannot be named because distance from the maternal object is a condition of speech. For example, the Ten Commandments are not really about the things named as prohibitions, but about what goes unnamed. The Commandments "regulate the distance between the subject and *das Ding* – insofar as that distance is precisely the condition of speech, insofar as the ten commandments are the condition of the existence of speech as such" (Lacan 1992, 69).

Ettinger, Bracha L. 2006a. Fascinance and the Girl-to-M/Other Matrixial Feminine Difference. In *Psychoanalysis and the Image*, ed. Griselda Pollock. Blackwell Publishing Ltd.

Ettinger, Bracha. 2006d. *The Matrixial Borderspace*, Theory out of Bounds. Vol. 28. University of Minnesota Press.

Haruki, Namiko. 2012. Ab-Sense of Existence in "The Ravishing of Lol Stein" by Marguerite Duras". *PSYART: A Hyperlink Journal for the Psychological Study of the Arts*, 5.

Lacan, Jacques. 1987. Homage to Marguerite Duras, on Le Ravissement de Lol V. Stein. In *Marguerite Duras*, translated by Peter Connor. City Lights Books.

Lacan, Jacques. 1992. *The Ethics of Psychoanalysis 1959–1960: The Seminar of Jacques Lacan*. Edited by Jacques-Alain Miller. Translated by Dennis Porter. Book VII. W. W. Norton & Company Inc.

Lacan, Jacques. 1998. *The Four Fundamental Concepts of Psychoanalysis, The Seminar of Jacques Lacan, Book XI*. Edited by Jacques-Alain Miller. Translated by Alan Sheridan. WW Norton & Company.

Lacan, Jacques. 2006e. Guiding Remarks for a Conversation on Female Sexuality. In *Écrits: The First Complete Edition in English*, translated by Bruce Fink. W.W. Norton & Company.

Lacan, Jacques. 2006g. The Subversion of the Subject and the Dialectic of Desire in the Freudian Unconscious. In *Écrits: The First Complete Edition in English*. Translated by Bruce Fink. W.W. Norton & Company.

Lacan, Jacques. 2011. The Seminar of Jacques Lacan: Book X: Anxiety: 1962–1963. Unpublished manuscript. Translated by Cormac Gallagher.

Rabaté, Jean-Michel. 2019. Falling in Love with Marguerite Duras. *Journal of the Circle for Lacanian Ideology Critique* 12:5–14.

7

Antigone and the "Jocasta Complex"

Bracha L. Ettinger and Jacques Lacan have both written on the Sophocles play *Antigone* and use it to articulate an ethics of psychoanalysis (Ettinger2000c, 2001, 2007, 2010, 2016; and Lacan 1992). For Lacan, Antigone's radical act of burying her brother Polynices in Theban soil despite the King's prohibition is an example of a true psychoanalytic act whereby the subject acts in accordance with their desire. The act cannot be understood in advance because it is particular to the subject and has no precedence in the law, culture, or history. Nor is it bound by the desire of the Other which, for Lacan, concerns the Symbolic. For Lacan, the radical act is not only the basis of a psychoanalytic ethic, but it reveals "to us the line of sight that defines desire" (247). Antigone's desire to forego her own life to ensure her brother's burial involves a transgression of a mortal limit. It is, as Lacan explains in *The Ethics of Psychoanalysis*, death-bound. From an analytic perspective, Antigone's act involves something akin to the end of analysis whereby there is a subjective destitution accompanied by a loss in being; that is, a coming to terms with one's own life predicament and mortality.

While Ettinger agrees that the transgression is deadly, Antigone's radical act is, for her, a transgression within to the Feminine dimension that

S. L. Cavanagh, *Bracha L. Ettinger and Jacques Lacan*, The Palgrave Lacan Series,
https://doi.org/10.1007/978-3-032-23293-9_7

must be understood in relation to her mother, Jocasta. Unlike Lacan who understands the psychoanalytic act as a relinquishing of the subject's being in relation to the Other's desire, the Other being first and foremost the mother in the Lacanian paradigm, the Ettingerian position is quite different. Ettinger's position is that the mother-Jocasta cannot be relinquished without harm being done to the mother–daughter borderlinking in the matrixial web. She views Antigone's radical defiance of the King as driven by a primal need to respect the integrity of the matrixial web and to do justice to the no-longer present presence of the mother Jocasta, who, like Antigone, takes her own life. For Ettinger, Antigone suffers from an irreparable tear from the mother and her kin due not only to the unimaginable edict issued by Creon, but by the incestuous transgression committed by Oedipus, her brother and father and Jocasta as mother.

One of Ettinger's major contributions to feminist psychoanalytic readings of the play is to show how Antigone's radical act is inspired by a Feminine-matrixial ethic whereby she cannot be without Jocasta or her brother (as *non-I*) and partner-in-difference. Ettinger develops a conceptualization of the Jocasta-with-Antigone matrixial web (2010, 1) that is occluded in Lacan's explication of the drama. Antigone's radical act illuminates what lies in excess of the King's rule: specifically a Feminine stratum of difference beyond the law, the word and the Lacanian signifier.

In this chapter, I outline Ettinger's interpretation of *Antigone* with attention to her critique of Lacan. For Ettinger, Lacan's emphasis on beauty, the limit, and the second-death in *Seminar VII* obfuscates a Feminine-axis of difference which can be understood in relation to the sub-Symbolic (matrixial-field). She claims that Lacan folds the matrixial into the phallic-castration stratum. More specifically, Ettinger argues that he folds the signifier "womb" into the phallic axis of difference, thereby foreclosing on the matrixial-Feminine dimension. The problem, as Ettinger understands it, is that Lacan does not give us a way to articulate the transgression with-in-to the Feminine of relevance to the matrixial. In so doing, Lacan misses what Ettinger calls a "supplementary value to the figure of the brother" (2000c, 193) and reinforces the idea of the "unexchangeable One" (2000c, 193; 2010, 13) which is only true in the phallic stratum. This is to say that the m/Other and the Feminine dimension are, for Ettinger, subsumed into the phallic axis of difference in Lacan's discourse.

In what follows, I provide a brief outline of the play and discuss the spectre of death, the limit, and the Other in the Lacanian analysis alongside the Ettingerian critique of Lacan with special attention to what she calls the Jocasta Complex inclusive of the two modes of incest haunting Antigone. I show how Ettinger's conceptualization of the Jocasta Complex is an important supplement to Lacan's writing on *Antigone*, but not at odds with his formulation of the m/Other as central to the drama.

Antigone

Feminist scholars have labored over the question of Antigone and her radical defiance of Creon, her King and uncle (e.g., see Butler 2002; Kristeva 2010; Irigaray 2010; Söderbäck 2010; Sjöholm 2004). Antigone's motivation for the burial of her brother, Polynices, in disregard of the King's edict has also been the source of great philosophical debate from Hegel to Lacan.

While we might dismiss her actions as examples of martyrdom, sacrificing her own life for the dignity of Polynices's corpse (and sacrificing her own well-being to care for her exiled father/brother in *Oedipus in Colonus*), feminists have tended to examine her transgression as not only fiercely independent and active, but as having conveyed something about feminine ethics and difference: specifically how feminine ethics and difference contravene or are irreconcilable with the state.

For example, Judith Butler (2002) and Julia Kristeva (2010) have both weighed in on the ethical significance of *Antigone*. As Butler explains, due to the Oedipal incestuous transgression, Antigone's life is already outside kinship norms and gender mores (Butler 2002), leaving her in a place of symbolic exile. In Julia Kristeva's assessment, Antigone cannot be subject to political justice because she is beyond human norms due to the incestuous legacy of Oedipus (2010, 217). Both daughter and sister to Oedipus who famously kills his father and marries his mother, Antigone lives in the shadow of a patricidal and incestuous transgression. Her mother, Jocasta, takes her own life (after learning the truth of her sinful marriage to her son), her brothers take each other's lives in battle over their father's legacy and kingdom, Haemon (Antigone's fiancé) dies by a sword meant for his father (the King) and she, Antigone, disowns her sister, Ismene, for refusing to join her in giving their brother burial rites in Theban soil.[1] Even Creon says that Antigone worships death. While Polynices is dead yet unburied, Antigone is ear-marked to die while still alive by the King.

Antigone's non-place in Thebes is brutally symbolized by her uncle, King Creon, who refuses to dignify her brother Polynices with a proper burial and threatens Antigone with death. For Creon, Polynices as an enemy of the state. He made war with Thebes and was willing to kill his brother, Eteocles, in competition for the Oedipal throne, rule of the Theban Kingdom. Brothers born of the same womb are diametrically opposed in battle and die. Antigone's fiancé Hemon remains loyal to his betrothed and dies by his own sword while trying to slay his father, Creon. Death looms large in the drama. Consequently, the question of entombment is what drives Antigone as it relates to her brother Polynices who was, even before his death, exiled by the state. Antigone chooses to honor Polynices's corpse by burying him (twice) in Theban soil. She does this knowing full well that she will lose her life and ultimately her cousin and fiancé Hemon, son of the King. Tiresias, the Theban seer and blind prophet, manages to persuade the King to spare Antigone's life. But the abrogation comes too late: Antigone hangs herself in a cave (tomb).

The Spectre of Death, the Limit, and the Other in Lacan

The incestuous legacy of Oedipus and Jocasta engulfs Antigone and she is living between what Lacan calls "two deaths," a death in life as distinct from a physical death. For him, she establishes *herself* at the limit (1992, 278). Lacan says, of Antigone, that she exists in the "place [where she is born] between two deaths" (226): one death to come due to the King's

[1] Bonnie Honig (2011) argues that the first unlawful burial of Polynices may have been done by Ishmene, not Antigone. If this is true, Antigone does not really disown her sister but acts in her defense by assuming responsibility for both burials.

edict, and the second death due, in part, to the Oedipal (incestuous) transgression that gives her life no coherent place in kinship structures. In this way, she lives what Lacan calls a second death (a phrase he takes from Marquis de Sade's 1795, *Philosophy in the Bedroom*), which is a death in life. As Lacan notes, Antigone enters the non-space of the second death, which is living while knowing that one has been condemned to death not only symbolically but literally. As such, Lacan positions Antigone between two deaths: she lives death in life and reveals an unrelenting death drive. In the play, Antigone says: "I have no home on earth and none below, not with the living, not with the breathless dead" (Sophocles 1984, 103). To her brother-father Oedipus, she says, "Your marriage murders mine, your dying drags me down to death alive" (103).

The hallmark of a tragic hero, for Lacan, is their movement beyond the limit established by the structure. But Ettinger contends, as I will explain below, that the Lacanian limit is the limit of the symbolic only. From the perspective of the matrixial, there is a sub-symbolic where Antigone's act is not only death bound but life-generating and about the future. Antigone's survival, bound up as it is with Polynices's burial (the family crypt), is beyond the phallic limit but firmly within the matrixial where, Ettinger contends, the Feminine ethic is about the future and knowing that life precedes one's own existence. Matrixial ethics cannot be symbolized by words, but they operate through co-affecting and aesthetic fields in Ettinger's formulation. Building upon Lévinas, Ettinger explains that the Feminine is the "irreducible difference inside subjectivity: precisely what makes it human" (2006, 190). The irreducible difference inside subjectivity concerns the mother as first and primary Other. For Ettinger, Lacan does not pay due respect to the centrality of the mother. Nor does he consider how the death of Jocasta effects the daughter-Antigone.

Ettinger reminds us that Jocasta consummates the Oedipal-legacy of incest that is Antigone's birthright. Moreover, she abandons Antigone in death by suicide. It follows that Antigone must also be mourning her mother, Jocasta, along with her brother and nephew, Polynices. The King's denial of burial rites to Polynices is doubly hurtful because it not only condemns her brother-nephew to the underworld but also disrespects her mother, Jocasta, as progenitor and ancestor. It is not death that drives a knife in the matrixial web but the "passage to bestiality that threatens to blow up and explode this sphere altogether into separate pieces" (205). Left unburied and open to the birds and swine, Polynices's corpse is brutally exposed to the elements. By denying Polynices his burial rites Antigone's sibling-nephew is reduced to the level of the non-human animal and Jocasta, as mother (along with her father-brother Oedipus), the progenitor(s) of a monstrosity.

Did Lacan Forget the m/Other?

While Ettinger's writing on Antigone emphasizes the vitally important role of the m/Other in the Sophocles drama, we should remember that Lacan also knows that the m/Other is central. He may be critiqued for not elaborating upon what he, in other seminars, calls the law of the mother in the tragedy.[2] But Lacan does not misunderstand the role of the m/Other in *Antigone* or, indeed, in psychoanalysis more generally. Lacan, like Ettinger, knows that the m/Other is at the origin of Antigone's desire and that the mother's position in the drama is central. In fact, Lacan writes in relation to Antigone that the "desire of the mother is the origin of everything. The desire for the mother is the founding desire of the whole structure" (Lacan 1992, 283).

What differs is the way each psychoanalyst narrates Antigone's relation to her familial others/Others. Ettinger is interested in the traumatic traces bequeathed to Antigone by Jocasta and their dispersal through her radical act. "What is at stake here is the *psychic site* of the trauma of the other with-in myself reached by force of the brother's alliance with the *I*" (Ettinger 2010, 13). Likewise, Lacan contends that Antigone's act is linked to her brother Polynices but he does not elaborate upon the linkage to the m/Other which is why Ettinger's critical supplement is so important. Lacan seems to focus on the specificity of the sibling relation because it is, as Antigone's speeches insist upon, the reason she will take her life; she can never have another brother.[3] Lacan writes: "The Greek

[2] See Morel (2018) for a discussion of the Law of the Mother in Lacan.

[3] The fact that Antigone can never have another mother is, interestingly, not addressed in her speeches.

term that expresses the joining of oneself to a brother or sister recurs throughout the play, and it appears right away in the first line when Antigone is speaking to Ismene" (1992, 255). Apart from this reference, Lacan does not say much else about Ismene (and nor does Ettinger). But Ettinger is on point when she insists upon the way Antigone's radical act is about the m/other. Specifically, she writes that the "Transgression is thus fatally linked to and binding with death-drive, incest, and the desire of the mother" (Ettinger 2010, 12).

Other feminists, like Judith Butler, have accused Lacan of seeming to be unconcerned with "how certain kinds of lives, precisely by virtue of the historical drama that is theirs, are relegated to the limits of the ineffaceable" (Butler 2002, 50). While it may be true that Lacan's writing is not about what sociologists call social justice, trauma studies, or feminism in the Theban city, it is more accurate to say that Lacan's psychoanalytic ethic is focused upon the psychic struggle Antigone negotiates in life (as opposed to her actual death). For him, the symbolic death is not about gender or the precarity of life as theorized by Butler (2004a), but about Antigone's positioning within the Symbolic structure. Lacan is, nevertheless, concerned not only about what Butler calls the precarity of life (2004a) and the ungrievability of those whose lives do not seem to matter (Butler 2016), but with Antigone's non-being in life: her second death. It is difficult to understand why Lacan would choose *Antigone* as a case study for an ethics of psychoanalysis if he was not interested in the limits constituted by her historically significant predicament.

In fact, Lacan is preoccupied by the question of what it means to live when one is condemned literally and symbolically to death. He is, in other words, concerned with Antigone's *being* in the Symbolic and with the subjective limit of death (as distinct from a biological death). This formulation is not unlike the Heideggerian formulation of a *being* toward death.[4] For Lacan, this Symbolic death is a subjective limit to the possible; it is unsurpassable and historically structured by the subject's being which, of course, includes the patriarchal structure (as part of the Symbolic). Lacan refers to the historical component of death as that

[4] Lacan's formulation of the second death differs from Heidegger's 'being-unto-death' insofar as it involves anxiety (2011, 8).

"which manifests itself in an inverted form in repetition. This is the "dead person [*le mort*] subjectivity takes as its partner in the triad instituted by its mediation in the universal conflict of *Philia,* love, and *Neikos*, strife" (Lacan 2006l, 262).[5]

Lacan also speaks of death in life as a "zone" and, more specifically, a zone that incarnates the "effect of beauty on desire" (Lacan 1992, 248). This is the image that Lacan calls the splendor of Antigone. He tells us that the "phenomenon of the beautiful…[is] the limit of the second death" (260). The concept of the limit is significant in Lacanian discourse because it is what one finds beyond the signifier. Lacan wonders about the "fate of a life that is about to turn into certain death, a death lived by anticipation, a death that crosses over into the sphere of life, a life that moves into the realm of death" (248). He concedes that there is "meaning at the limit, but there is nobody to signify it" (184–185). Those who go beyond the limits of the Symbolic are, for him, living a desire that can only mean death. In Lacanian terms, we enter a second death when we cross a limit for too long. For Lacan, Antigone exists at the limit (248). This limit is a living death. Indeed, Antigone says, "I gave myself to death, long ago, so I might serve the dead" (Sophocles 1984, 88). Antigone is foisted into what Lacan calls a living death which includes knowledge of pending death in life.

Indeed, the spectre of death overshadows the play. If we read the trilogy backward, begin with *Oedipus at Colonus*, proceed to *Oedipus the King*, and end with *Antigone*, we witness the actual death of almost every character in the House of Oedipus. Ettinger contends that what is so horrific about the story of Antigone, from a matrixial point of view, is the "matrixial loss by definitive cut…in this psychical zone, a horror beyond its scope" (2000c, 198). The horror is not only about the loss of Jocasta and the indignity to her brother's corpse but about what both do to the Feminine axis of difference in the familial web. While the Feminine axis of difference is not the same as what Lacan calls the second death, its obfuscation in the phallic can be compared to an erasure or denial of

[5] Lacan suggests that what is negated in discourse may be caused by death. "For the negativity of discourse, insofar as it brings into being that which is not, refers us to the question of what nonbeing, which manifests itself in the symbolic order, owes to the reality of death" (2006l, 316).

being in the Symbolic. Ettinger does not make this claim but both psychoanalysts are, in my reading, grappling with a Symbolic erasure of epic significance to the subject.

Ettinger seems to be indicating that the matrixial must be inscribed when she stresses the importance of honoring Polynices burial rites and Lacan focuses on the radical importance of Antigone's speeches which are original and unprecedented. For Antigone, Polynices must be buried because the burial functions like an inscription that is also a borderlinking. A borderlinking occurs in what Lacan calls the Real and involves what Ettinger calls an aggregated subjectivity (not reducible to intersubjectivity). In one of her most important articles on *Antigone*, Ettinger's (2010) thesis relating to borderlinking in the Feminine-matrixial is developed through an analysis of what Judith Butler calls kinship trouble and gender trouble in her now classic book titled *Antigone's Claim* (2002). A brief detour through Ettinger's analysis and extension of Butler's work on the play will help us to understand the Feminine-matrixial at stake in Antigone's plight.

Gender Trouble and the Matrixial

For Ettinger, *Antigone* is a feminist classic because it gives us a way to understand the protagonist's devotion to her brother *and* the centrally important role of Jocasta, as mother, in the tragedy. But Ettinger claims that both Antigone and her brother-nephew, Polynices, signify more than individual-phallic subjects. Responding to Judith Butler's (2002) argument in *Antigone's Claim* that gender and kinship orders are undone in the Sophocles tragedy and that, by the end of the play, Antigone has "taken the place of nearly every man in her family" (62),[6] Ettinger considers what she calls "hidden [matrixial] potentialities" (Ettinger 2010, 1) in Butler's astute analysis. While Butler asks important questions about what network of gender and kinship relations might make life on the

[6] Consider that Antigone's gender is masculinized in the play. Oedipus refers to his 'daughter' Antigone as a son; the King insists he will not be 'unmanned' by Antigone; and the chorus refers to her as 'manly.'

margins of cultural intelligibility representable (and thus livable), Ettinger asks a comparable set of questions about the status of the m/Other (Jocasta) and the Feminine in the phallic stratum. Like the gender and kinship trouble that falls outside Theban norms, the Ettingerian Feminine lacks (phallic) recognition. We may even say that the Feminine exists in a state of exception. It is not that gender variance stands in for the matrixial or that matrixiality is, by definition, gender variant, but rather that confusion *in the play* about gender may be metonymically tied to the Feminine-matrixial foreclosed in the city of Thebes ruled by the patriarchal King.

Was Antigone insisting upon legal recognition of a Feminine law associated with what Ettinger calls the matrixial? As Butler notes, to insist upon the "legality of what does not exist and of what is unconscious…some form of demand that the unconscious necessarily makes on law, that which marks the limit and condition of law's generalizability" (2002, 33) is, ultimately, what Antigone does. Can this demand be understood in relation to the Feminine-matrixial? Butler says that the unconscious law "leaves only an incommunicable trace, an enigma of another possible order" (39), but does not describe this order as Feminine (or masculine-phallic). While Ettinger's Feminine-matrixial is not reducible to gender, the Feminine-matrixial taps into an otherness that Ettinger calls Feminine—not in a demographic or identitarian sense but rather, as a condition of becoming that recalls and is predicated on a relation, Real and Imaginary, to natal female sexual reproductive capacity. The Ettingerian Feminine is not an axis of difference specific to natal female subjects, however. This Other (Feminine) sexual difference is available to everyone regardless of natal sex, gender identity or sexual orientation as discussed in previous chapters.

Butler claims that Antigone figures as the law's unconscious and as such remains opaque to it. She also speculates that Antigone's refusal to abide by the orders of the King, as representative of the state, is not only an instance of feminist or, possibly, gender queer rebellion, but a commentary on her no-place in kinship structures and by extension the polis. Due to Oedipus's formative incestuous transgression (in the phallic/paternal), Antigone occupies a range of un-authorized familial positions: she is daughter and sister to her father/brother (Oedipus); sister and aunt to her nephew/brother (Polyneices), and daughter and granddaughter to her mother/grandmother (Jocasta).[7] Butler's point is that Antigone is not only a "woman" but in "some sense she is also a man" (2010, 136). The masculine version of Antigone is "Antigonus" which literally means worthy of or, existing in place of, one's parents. Antigone effectively becomes not the man but the "men" in the family. In fact, Creon wonders if she is a man and Antigone is called a "man" (*aner*) in the play. She is, as Butler suggests, a brother in/by confusion.

What Butler refers to as kinship trouble and gender trouble is, for Ettinger, an "unexpected site of resistance and co-emergence" (2010, 1) relevant to the matrixial. The slippages so well noted by Butler between gender, identity, and kinship positions in the drama indexes, for Ettinger, a non-phallic axis of difference where subjects are bound to others in difference. This is not to say that gender variance is, by definition, matrixial, but that gender variance may stand-in to represent something relevant to the matrixial that is illegible in the Theban Kingdom, and thus occluded in the phallic Symbolic. The confusion of gender, kinship norms, and generation in *Antigone* stands in for an unlivable foreclosure of the m/Other in Ettinger's interpretation. In relation to Butler's thesis regarding gender, recognition, and kinship disorder, Ettinger writes: "My perspective leads me to infuse this confusion with the Place of the m/Other and as *Sister-daughter*, and to consider the confusion of generations with the foreclosure of the m/Other, adding, thus, a matrixial Eros to Antigone's search for forms of love" (Ettinger 2010, 16). In other words, Ettinger adds another dimension to the Butlerian analysis of gender and kinship disorder that involves questions about "place" and "time." The "place" of the m/Other and the "time" of borderlinking in the matrixial are both relevant. "With an *Antigone as Place of the Brother* qua *Place of Loss* that does carry within it the *delphys*, the Place of the m/Other, even Oedipus is no longer so Oedipal; even Oedipus can function as a pole in a co-poietic string, and each son is *also* a Daughter in a matrixial sense" (16). Ettinger is, in my interpretation, concerned with what becomes of the

[7] In her essay "Antigone: Limit and Horizon" Kristeva (2010) notes that the mother Jocasta is the "*only one* who persists in her own identity because she is the mother of everyone, including Oedipus; while Oedipus, the father, is himself also the child of *this* mother, but not the only one, since he is not the father of Jocasta" (219).

matrixial elements of the human subject in a phallic order that is not only sexist and cis-heteronormative as Butler would agree, but unable to grapple with the Feminine-matrixial elements of being.

What Antigone avows and approaches with unwavering desire is a "difference in the Real" (2000c, 206), a traumatic encounter with the other and the other's Other. For Ettinger, Antigone's transgression gives us sub-knowledge of the Feminine involving, among other things, death and borderlinking. This may call to mind Lacan's complaint that female psychoanalysts have done little to unearth the secrets of the Other jouissance. The question remaining to be asked: Is this Feminine-matrixial interpretation of the drama wholly distinct from Lacan's reading of Antigone's plight and transgression? My contention is that Ettinger offers a matrixial formulation of the Other and the Real that corresponds to Lacan's teachings. While Ettinger's interpretation pays greater attention to the role m/Other in the drama than Lacan does, both scholars know that Antigone is driven by something more than the law of the father symbolized by the King.

The Lacanian Other and the Feminine-matrixial

Consider that Lacan does not choose Oedipus but, rather, Antigone to develop his position on psychoanalytic ethics. Lacan finds in Antigone's courageous, yet brutal, act, an ethic for psychoanalysis. In his view, Antigone's ethic should not be confused with saintliness or martyrdom. In fact, Lacan underscores the aggressiveness of the ethical act. In his discussion of the heroine, Lacan refers to her as "inhuman" and "inflexible" (1992, 263), as "fierce" (265), and "savage" (278). Antigone "feels neither fear nor pity" (258). She chooses to honor Polynices's corpse knowing full well that she will lose her life and ultimately her cousin and fiancé Haemon (son of the Creon). Lacan is struck by Antigone's refusal to yield, by what some have called her "idiocy" (265): the "unshakable, unyielding position of Antigone is fixed" (279). The way she "freezes" the signifier, the "it" of the Real, is what occupies Lacan's imagination. He is concerned with the ineffaceable mark of her act without reference to "content, to whatever good or evil Polynices may have done, or to whatever he may be subjected to" (279).

Ettinger's suggestion that Lacan does not grapple with the matrixial elements of the human subject is, in my reading, questionable. Lacan knows that what drives Antigone to act is not about the law of the land, Creon (the King), or even the Symbolic. He contends that Antigone is driven by her *Até*, a mortal limit which concerns the field of the Other, a field that, Lacan reminds us, "does not belong to Creon, [but] is on the other hand, the place where Antigone is situated" (277). The *Até* is not unlike the Feminine-matrixial dimension theorized by Ettinger, even if Lacan does not call it Feminine per se. Let us recall that *Até* is an ancient Greek word referring to a Goddess who acts upon a fatal and reckless blindness. It can also be used to refer to that which harms or misleads. Lacan is fascinated by Antigone's unyielding certainty, but also by what drives her beyond the limit of her *Até*. He says that something beyond the limits of "*Até* has become Antigone's good, namely, a good that is different from everyone else's, that she goes toward [*Até*]" (270).

Furthermore, Lacan writes that Antigone's beauty radiates from a place that is an "intermediary between two fields that are symbolically differentiated' (248). It is not entirely clear what Lacan means by these two fields, except that they are, like the phallic and what Ettinger calls the Feminine-matrixial, symbolically differentiated. But we might find a clue in Lacan's conception of beauty. Beauty is, for Lacan, a radical negativity that radiates and resides at the limit. Antigone's beauty is a splendor deriving from the limit. Lacanian "beauty" is not an aesthetic ideal. He regards Antigone's beauty in a Kantian sense (not as an ideal). He also, following Kant, calls beauty "sublime" (286). It veils our relation to the *Thing* (*das Ding*) which Lacan later calls *object a*.[8] The *Thing/object a* stands in for the m/Other's unnameable desire. The object-a cause of desire is, for Lacan, not only about the m/Other but about the beautiful which acts as a barrier between life and death. It acts like a cloak concealing "all possible

[8] Beauty camouflages a void structuring desire. Like an empty vase, beauty gives contour to the void. Lacan evokes the empty center and, more precisely, the curvature of a vase to capture the essence of the void in and around which desire circles. Beauty is best understood as a 'pulsion, an insistence and a repetition behind which or beyond which there is only a void' (Freeland 2013, 150).

fantasms of human desire" (298). It is an interface that functions more like a mirage than a subjective attribute.

In relation to Antigone whose life was marked for death at the time of her birth, Lacan refers to a beauty effect that "derives from the relationship of the hero to the limit" (286). This is a limit that Antigone is born into and must negotiate in life. Her life exists at a limit marked by death. Jouissance is also a limit in Lacanian psychoanalysis and involves a line of no return. Lacan is not only concerned with why Antigone cannot live due to the specific conditions of her birth, but with the centrally important question of her desire and death-bound jouissance. What interests Lacan is the way a "human being is defined by desire's insatiable *pulsion* toward what it cannot attain" (Freeland 2013, 164). When Lacan writes that Antigone is "desire of death as such" (1992, 282), he doesn't mean that she is suicidal. He means that she is pure desire, above and beyond the Law.

According to Lacan, Antigone's desire is an inhuman transgression of the limit and involves a metamorphosis. He writes:

> The limit we have reached here is the one where the possibility of metamorphosis is located— metamorphosis that has come down through the centuries hidden in the works of Ovid and that regains its former vitality, its energy, during that turning point of European sensibility, the Renaissance, and bursts forth in the theater of Shakespeare. That is what Antigone is. (265)

Lacan's metamorphosis occurs when one reaches a limit imposed by the socio-Symbolic structure. Life at the limit inaugurates a change which Lacan, in his discussion of Antigone, calls a metamorphosis. The function of desire in drama is, for Lacan, to expose "what remains undetermined: in the collapse of the house of cards represented by tragedy, one thing may subside before another, and what one finds at the end when one turns the whole thing around may appear in different ways" (265). In her Lacanian reading of *Antigone*, Joan Copjec (2004) notes, for example, that the protagonist is not an intransigent character but a "figure of radical metamorphosis" (44).

Lacanian Limits, Thresholds, and the Ettingerian Metramorphosis

What Lacan does not theorize, in Ettinger's opinion, is the radiating presence of the Feminine "beyond-the-phallus" (Ettinger 2001, 83), and the way it involves a *metra*morphic transgression within to the Feminine dimension. Ettinger's notion of *metra*morphosis (2010, 13) is a matrixial variation of the Lacanian reference to metamorphosis. While Lacan's metamorphosis concerns the Symbolic and what lies beyond the limit (where the untouchable *Thing* resides), Ettinger's *metra*morphosis is a transgression within to the Feminine; a dimension of difference that recalls the m/Other.

For Ettinger, a metramorphosis is not structured by a limit but by an erotic threshold relevant to the matrixial borderspace. It has transformative potential but is also about co-fading. It is an intrapsychic and interpsychic phenomenon that is transindividual.[9] What Lacan calls a limit is, for Ettinger, a borderline. Through a metramorphic event-encounter there is a "joint awakening of unthoughtful-knowledge on the borderline, as well as an inscription of the encounter in traces that open a space in and along the borderline itself" (2006, 182). Event-encounters occur in shifting borderspaces where new ties and affective links are formed (and transgressed). Antigone is co-affected by, and co-emerging with-in-by, her brother and mother (as *non-I's*). Together, they are bound in matrixial terms and each partial-subject cannot be understood as one in a shared unconscious borderspace.

For Ettinger, the Lacanian limit is not a barrier; it is a threshold. As Ettinger writes, "the limit-frontier described by Lacan that separates the subject from the death drive cuts the subject also from feminine sexuality; and constructs the 'woman' as absent, and her 'rapport' as 'impossible,' and herself as out-of-existence significance" (2000a, 92). The limit Lacan postulates between life and death is, for Ettinger, a passage to the

[9] Ettinger writes that metramorphosis is a "process of intra-psychical and inter-psychical or trans-individual exchange, transformation and affective "communication", between/with-in several matrixial entities. It is a passage-lane through which affected events, materials and modes of becoming infiltrate and diversify onto non-conscious margins of the Symbolic through/by sub-symbolic webs" (2000c, 194).

matrixial sub-stratum whereby the *I* and the *non-I* are not individual (phallic) subjects, but borderlinked in matrixial terms. Borderlines are like thresholds, not limits. It should be remembered that the Ettingerian Feminine is predicated upon a "borderline coming-into-being" (2007, 119), a co-emergence that is both connective and differentiating. The co-emergence is subjectifying and copoietic. It involves a Feminine Eros particular to the matrixial. Through a metramorphic event-encounter, there is a "joint awakening of unthoughtful-knowledge on the borderline, as well as an inscription of the encounter in traces that open a space in and along the borderline itself" (2006, 182).

When we encounter a threshold, there is an encounter beyond the limit which is beautiful and sublime: beautiful and sublime because it functions like a "transport-station of trauma" (2000a, 92). The Lacanian limit is, for Ettinger, more like a hybrid margin. It involves an archaic trauma and jouissance, a jointness-in-difference with the archaic m/Other (95). In her discussion of matrixial desire, Ettinger (1997) notes that Feminine jouissance "sprouts not from a phantasy about sharing but from a border shareability in trauma and phantasy" (399). For Ettinger, "Feminine jouissance aspires to release itself and shape a feminine dimension of desire" (376). The archaic jouissance is linked to the Woman-m/Other who is not only an absence as Lacan contends, but a pre-absence and a phantasmic presence. As understood through the prism of Ettinger's matrixial, Antigone occupies a shared body-space that resonates and affects her as a co-emerging partial-subject in a suffocating familial web whereby there is no difference between kinship positions due to the Oedipus-Jocasta incestuous transgression.

In Ettingerian terms, Antigone channels the Feminine "beyond-the-phallus in the Other of culture" (Ettinger 2001, 83). Thus, Antigone's ethical act involves an inscription of the Feminine (Ettinger 2006) in the otherwise patriarchal landscape of the King. The heroine is guided by a matrixial precept and precedent as opposed to a phallic legal-code. Contra Lacan, Ettinger contends that what has to be wit(h)nessed—and what radiates with beauty—is the originary Feminine sexual rapport foundational to life, ethics, aesthetics, and futurity. This future, envisioned by Antigone, must not be understood in terms of death but rather in terms of Feminine Eros. This Eros is about borderlinking to Others and *non-I*'s in the matrixial web. For Ettinger, Antigone desires to register a matrixial incestual tear and this registration is about beauty, thresholds (not limits) and futurity.

Beauty is, for Ettinger, about the irreplaceable. It is co-affective, metramorphic, and ethical. Her formulation of beauty elaborates upon the Lacanian definition: "The effect of beauty results from the *rapport* of the subject to the horizon of life; from traversing to *the second death*" (Ettinger 2010, 11, emphasis in the original). What is beautiful, from a matrixial perspective, is the redistribution and re-affectation of traumatic trace encounters between partial-subjects in matrixial alliance (14).

Antigone lives on the limit where, as Ettinger writes, "her life is already lost, where she is already on the other side" (11). It is ex nihilo in Lacanian terms. This is a *being* on the limit is, for Lacan, beautiful because it is a "barrier that forbids access to a fundamental horror" (2006g, 654). What Lacan calls a fundamental horror is, for Ettinger, the matrixial time-space continuum where there *is*, to rewrite Lacan's formulation, an Other of the other. In effect, Ettinger challenges the Lacanian premise that there is no Other of the other. For Ettinger, there is an Other of the other in the matrixial dimension: generations that come before. Read through the lens of the matrixial, Antigone's radical act is not driven by a desire for severance or death, but for borderlinking to/with/in her m/Other. Ettinger contends that matrixial desire fuels a wish to close a gap between generations which is, ideally, sublimated into a Feminine ethic of com-passion. This com-passion is trans-sensitive insofar as it apprehends Others and *non-I*'s in the matrixial web. Antigone's position as partial-subject is transconnected to Polynices and Jocasta and it is from this borderspace that she speaks.

Ettinger develops a unique post-Lacanian feminist formulation of how the *I* is an Other. For Ettinger, the matrixial is another subjectivizing stratum where the m/Other is not the "Other but a border-Other, a becoming in-ter-with the Other, an im-pure becoming-between in jointness" (2001, 72). She contends that Antigone goes beyond the phallic-limit which is, for her, a threshold into an-Other (matrixial) borderspace in time. Ettinger is interested in Antigone's transgression as entry into a "surplus beyond" (2010, 13) where (and when) a metramorphic event-encounter reconfigures what counts, in the phallic prism, as a limit. As Ettinger explains:

> Transgression is still linked to death-drive, incest, and the desire of the mother, but this linkage itself is transformed, and with it, the meaning of each of these concepts in the feminine, where transgression is not a jump beyond a frontier, but an access to the surplus beyond, and thus, a transformation of the limits themselves with regard to the subject's affective access to the question of the death of 'her' other. (13)

The real issue for Ettinger involves not (only) the death of Polynices as "one" brother but also the death of the *non-I* in the *I*, which she elaborates in terms of the Jocaste-Antigone complex where trace-connections haunt Antigone.[10]

To summarize Ettinger's argument thus far: Antigone's desire involves an Other axis of difference bound to the Feminine-matrixial where our others and *non-I*'s are integral to our being. Ettinger postulates a Feminine Eros functioning at the level of the matrixial. Matrixial desire is not about amalgamation, aggressive incorporation or cuts, but co-emergence and differentiation in the borderlinking. The borderlinking does not generate signifiers (word-images) in Lacanian terms. Nor is it harmonious or utopic: it can be terrifying and traumatizing as Antigone discovers. Ettinger writes that the "desire to join-in-difference and differentiate-in-co-emergence with the Other…[involves] a joining with-in the other's trauma that echoes back to my archaic traumas" (2006, 147). Sharing by joining in difference and differentiating in co-emergence is profoundly unsettling insofar as it threatens us with mental disintegration and memory of oblivion. We are not, as Ettinger notes, "cut from lack", we "appear by disappearing" (147). This is, for Ettinger, a non-genital Feminine Eros that is nevertheless sexuating. Moreover, it is an Eros central to what Ettinger calls the Jocasta Complex.

[10] Like Ettinger, Butler is also suspicious of the claim that Antigone is only grieving her brother Polynices. Referring to Antigone's speech about the loss of her brother in his singularity, Butler writes: '[…] her insistence on the singularity of her brother, his radical irreproducibility, is belied by the mourning she fails to perform for her two other brothers [Oedipus and Eteocles], the ones she fails to reproduce publicly for us' (2002, 80).

The Jocasta Complex

Ettinger wonders why it is so difficult for people to understand Antigone's demand to bury her brother in Theban soil. The lack of compassion for Antigone's plight in the city of Thebes is not only a phallic oversight but also a structural negation of the Feminine dimension which is, as Ettinger explains, founded upon a denial of what she calls the Jocasta complex. In essence, she supplements the now-famous Oedipal Complex with the Jocasta complex.[11] Denial of the Jocasta complex is, for Ettinger, indicative of the extent to which psychoanalysis has ignored the significance of intrauterine experience (as explained in Chap. 2). Both Freud and Lacan believed that pre-birth experiences were unanalyzable and that subjectivity begins after birth. Ettinger contends that there are affective corpo-Real ties with-in/between the becoming-subject and the mother-to-be that predate the Oedipal complex (theorized by Freud) and the Lacanian signifier. For Ettinger, these co-affective ties are relevant to the clinic, even if they are not accessible by/through/in speech-acts. We are always more than One in the matrixial stratum. This is not to say that we do not exist as separate ethical subjects who must take legal responsibility for our acts. It is, rather, to say that we are always also aggregated subjects and thus, acting with/alongside Others (*non-I's*).

Ettinger contends that there is something in the position of girls-becoming-women and their relation to the m/Other (whether natal birth giving mother or maternal stand-in) that warrants a psychoanalytic term in itself, a "*principal within countertransference*" (2006, 109, original emphasis) that she names the Jocasta complex. Ettinger posits a theory of *besideness* as opposed to splitting or debinding in Kristevian terms (Cavanagh 2017).[12] The besideness posited by Ettinger involves a "*ratification* of her [the mother's] acts *without* any need for *identification* with her or rationalization of her acts" (Ettinger 2006, 109, original emphasis).

---

[11] See Matthew Besdine (1968) for an earlier psychoanalytic formulation of the Jocasta Complex.

[12] For Kristeva, Antigone makes a cut that paradoxically "regenerates the social bond…[by] going outside of the self – the limit state of an indivisible identity" (2010, 218). Ettinger takes issue with Kristeva's notion of 'debinding' which involves a cut from the m/Other. In Ettinger's estimation, Kristeva repeats a Lacanian problem relating to the obfuscation of the m/Other in her interpretation of the play (Cavanagh 2017).

Without a name for the dilemma of the mother as subject and the becoming-girl-woman-subject such as, for example, the "Jocasta Complex," we damage the Real of the mother/daughter (or mother/son) relationship: "the daughter blames the real mother for actual abandonment, and while languishing for perfect attunement with the Other and with the world, identifies with the turning of the womb into a tomb and engraving a psychic grave at the place of the originary string" (2010, 6).

The originary string is vital to the matrixial subject who is more than One. Ettinger contends that Antigone's transgression is with-in-to the Feminine and that the drama must be read from the perspective of the matrixial whereby characters are more than One. As explained in previous chapters, Ettinger posits a model of subjectivity as severality (the *I* with some others). In *Antigone*, each character carries a supplementary, trans-subjective value whereby they exist in relation to their *non-I*'s as partners in difference. The trans-subjective involves a Feminine transgression in Ettinger's terms. Her matrixial reading of the drama focuses upon a Transgression-within-to-the-Feminine which involves a borderlinking with the m/Other. Ettinger argues that this Feminine transgression is missing in Lacan's study of Antigone's radical act. In her view, he fails to understand Antigone's (matrixial) desire, the mortal limit as threshold (to the matrixial), and her radiant splendor (as involving beauty in the originary Feminine rapport). While Lacanian theory stresses the sexual non-rapport, there is, in Ettinger's interpretation of the drama, a non-genital sexual relation between Antigone and her m/Other as absent-presence. In order to account for matrixial trace connections to the m/Other, Ettinger contends that psychoanalysis needs a broader and more nuanced conception of the subject than the one modeled upon individual (Oedipal) subjectivity. Her oeuvre is an extensive mapping of this Other subjective (matrixial) dimension that is, as she writes, aggregated and dependent upon the m/Other.

Ettinger's (2010) formulation of the Jocasta Complex is a way to give conceptual form to the subject's being in relation to the m/Other. The Jocasta complex enables us to comprehend an Other (non-Oedipal) sexual difference evidenced in *Antigone*. It is a Feminine difference that involves both a sub-subjective field (involving an aggregated subjectivity) and a trans-subjective field (involving uncognized *non-I*'s and others).

The sub-subjective dimension can be accessed through self-fragilization when, for example, we relinquish identitarian borders or, in Antigone's case, normative kinship positions. We risk fragmentation and what Butler (2004b) might call "coming undone" to meet an Other partial-subject in a shared borderspace. We may experience "dispersal and loss of the self" (Ettinger 2009, 21) in the sub-subjective psychic space. For Ettinger, this is what Antigone felt as she lived not only under the prospect of death, but with the knowledge that her brother's unburied corpse lay open and exposed. Antigone was dealing with what we might, to use Ettinger's terms, call the "shock of corporeality," mortality and co-implication *with* and *in* the Other.

Incest and the Matrixial

In Ettinger's interpretation, Antigone is not only tormented by the Oedipal transgression, but by Jocasta's transgression which effectively combines two forms of incest: one that is traumatizing and the other that is essential to life. In Ettinger's reading, *Antigone* (as one play in the Sophocles trilogy) dramatizes the difference between the two. The Oedipal complex, as theorized by Freud and countless psychoanalysts to follow, is focused upon what Ettinger calls phallic incest: sexual acts between people of a shared bloodline. This form of incest is subject to cultural taboo and legal prohibition. The second kind of incest involves pregnancy and birth. It involves Antigone and Jocasta (who do not have sex) and is, as such, primary, unavoidable, and generative. It occurs in the womb. It links the mother-to-be and the subject-to-be in a "shared matrixial Real…pre-subjectivity is saturated by transjective resonance, [where] trans-generational transmission…occurs by co-emerging with the archaic m/Other" (Ettinger 2010, 5). Life depends upon it. *Becoming* is ultimately linked to an incestuous transgression in/with/by the-mother-to-be. Matrixial incest cannot be outlawed although it is subject to repression. It does not generate structures of prohibition although it lacks cultural value and, as Ettinger contends, incorrectly reduced to fusion and symbiosis.

Ettinger claims that matrixial desire fuels a wish to close a gap between generations that is impossible (outside the womb) and ultimately (ideally) sublimated into a Feminine ethic of com-passion. This com-passion is trans-sensitive insofar as it apprehends Others and *non-I*'s in the matrixial web. Matrixial desire lacks value and intelligibility in the phallic stratum. By burying Polynices, Antigone is also burying her mother. The heroine is grieving the unsymbolized dimensions of the maternal connection which are incestuous, traumatic, and multiple.

Another way to think about the two forms of incest that Antigone inherits is in relation to what Abraham and Torok (1994) call a psychic crypt. As Ettinger explains, "Antigone is also heir to an encrypted maternal enigma she cannot access without sharing with a *non-I*. She carries traces of this enigma" (2010, 5). This is to say that Antigone is heir to both maternal and phallic incestuous transgressions. Jocasta abandons Oedipus and in so doing colludes in "paternal infanticide impulses" (6) even as she tries to save her son from Laius by abandoning him to a shepherd when he was a baby. But by a second, "supplementary abandonment, she disappeared to her daughters" (6) by suicide. The mother's transgressions become psychic traces passed down to Antigone through maternal and paternal lines or, in Ettinger's words, through affective traces and *a-links*. The ethical impossibilities of Jocasta's situation as mother, as partner in Oedipal and paternal-infanticidal transgressions, may be extreme and unlawful but, nevertheless, resonate, for generations of people spellbound by the tragedy.

Ettinger' formulation of the Jocasta Complex gives us a way to understand the traumatic traces bequeathed to Antigone by Jocasta and their dispersal through the daughter's radical act. "What is at stake here is the *psychic site* of the trauma of the other with-in myself reached by force of the brother's alliance with the *I*" (13). What Ettinger calls the "Jocaste-with-Antigone matrixial web" (1) has been ruptured. Through a matrixial alliance, Antigone carries a transitive trauma inherited from Jocasta that can only be put to rest by burying the family psychic crypt (Abraham and Torok 1994).

Ettinger claims that when the matrixial elements of the subject are negated or erased the mother becomes a "ready-made monster" and the womb is foreclosed as a non-place (Ettinger 2010). The actual mother becomes a scapegoat or rendered insignificant and the mother-in-the-daughter as *non-I* is damned. As Ettinger summarizes, the "foreclosure of transcrypted traces, unaccessed for lack of terms to render them intelligible, makes this side of the transmitted scenario non-livable. The *real trauma* of the *non-I*, carried by her body, becomes an unconscious active *phantasmatic agent* in the *I*" (Ettinger 2010, 7). It follows that by burying Polynices Antigone is also doing justice to her mother and the unsymbolized dimensions of the maternal connection laced with loss and incestuous trauma. Jocasta and Antigone's psychical struggles are inter-implicated and co-affecting. For Ettinger, Antigone's link to her mother is primary, Oedipalization and (phallic) sexuality are secondary. She writes, for "Jocaste-with-Antigone: a yearning beating searches for the resonance emanating from the struggle for meaning-creation over a transcrypted bleeding, a lamenting womb – as time-space of sharing of m/Other with brothers – where fascinance and compassion resonate in com-passion beyond different times and places" (11).

Ettinger concludes that Antigone would rather end her own life than bear a cut in her matrixial web represented by her brother's unburied corpse. She persuasively argues that Antigone transgresses the law of the King in order to preserve her maternal link to Jocasta (as mother). Antigone knows that matrixial linkages must not be annihilated by the Other's tyrannical jouissance, symbolized by Creon. Polynices must be seen to have existed through the enactment of a state-sanctioned burial. His *being* as Other is bound up with multiple Others (as partial-subjects) in the House of Oedipus.

Conclusion

One of Ettinger's major claims is that the Feminine dimension of being cannot remain in a state of exception and thus foreclosed in psychoanalysis and in culture more generally. This is not to say that we do not exist as separate subjects in the (phallic) Symbolic, but that we are always aggregated (partial-subjects), more than One in the matrixial stratum. The Other in the *I* must be analyzed in a transjective sense to deal with shared trauma in the Feminine matrixial. As Ettinger explains, the "human body with-in this [matrixial] borderspace is not the last barrier from the Other-beyond, but the *passage* to an other" (2010, 12). We can no longer appeal to Oedipus and his interpersonal drama without attending to Antigone and Jocasta, as partners in difference, in the family romance and in culture at large. As Butler agrees, Antigone's trauma is post-Oedipal (2002, 57). She is his descendant and as a descendent, she is re-living a past drama bequeathed to her by an Other, but in a changed form.

Despite Ettinger's important contributions to post-Lacanian feminist thought, her contention that the m/Other can be signified in an expanded symbolic, when due attention is given to the Feminine dimension, is not inconsistent with the stress Lacan places upon the position of the brother-Polynices. Lacan suggests that the desire for recognition sought by Antigone is not really a question of legal recognition of the person Polynices. It is desire for symbolic recognition of his position *as* brother. Because there is more than one character that occupies the position of brother and, also because Oedipus (as father) is also brother, there is a lack of symbolic differentiation. In Lacan's estimate, Antigone's desire is not to die, but to lend symbolic support to the position of brother. She seeks to strengthen the Symbolic position of her kin. This is what Lacan means when he says that Antigone loves the "pure being" of her brother. What Antigone wants is authorization for her brother's very being, which will, by extension, help inscribe her own being as a subject in the Symbolic. In so doing, Antigone is the "guardian of the being of the criminal as such" (Lacan 1992, 283). No one else in her family is left to "assume the [crime that is Jocasta's desire] and the validity of the crime apart from Antigone" (283). Lacan is not making a moral claim here. He is underlying Antigone's function in the incestual and patricidal familial structure.

Antigone's radical act is, for Ettinger, less about the position of the brother as criminal and the Oedipal legacy than it is about enabling life and a Feminine Eros (although she concedes that Antigone's desire is death-bound). Ettinger writes that the "frontier that separates the human being from death converges with the frontier that separates the human being from the feminine" (Ettinger 2010, 12). Antigone accesses a surplus beyond a phallic frontier (or life limit) where one's desire and jouissance is in the borderlinking. Antigone is co-affected by, and co-emerging with-in-by, her brother and mother (as *non-I*'s). She lays Polynices to rest with her very being, not in a sacrificial way, but in an effort to bury and mourn a traumatic familial crypt. In Ettingerian vernacular, she wit(h) nesses her Other in compassionate hospitality and knows that there is a future without her. Antigone does not only reveal a radiant-splendor bound-up in death (as theorized by Lacan), but the partial-subject's relation to the m/Other. This latter relation is, for Ettinger, repressed in the phallic stratum. It needs to be articulated through art and through what she calls "care-full com-passion and faith-full wit(h)nessing – through *communicaring*" (14).

Bibliography

Abraham, Nicolas, and Maria Torok. 1994. *The Shell and the Kernel: Renewals of Psychoanalysis, Volume 1*. Translated by Nicholas T. Rand. Vol. 1. University of Chicago Press. WorldCat.

Besdine, Matthew. 1968. The Jocasta Complex, Mothering and Genius, Part I. *Psychoanalytic Review* (New York) 55 (2): 259. Periodicals Archive Online (1310161122).

Butler, Judith. 2002. *Antigone's Claim: Kinship between Life & Death*, The Wellek Library Lectures. Columbia University Press.

Butler, Judith. 2004a. *Precarious Life: The Powers of Mourning and Violence*. Verso.

Butler, Judith. 2004b. *Undoing Gender*. 1st ed. Taylor & Francis Group. https://doi.org/10.4324/9780203499627.

Butler, Judith. 2010. Promiscuous Obedience. In *Feminist Readings of Antigone*, ed. Fanny Söderbäck, 1st ed. State University of New York Press.

Butler, Judith. 2016. *Frames of War: When is Life Grievable?* Verso Books.

Cavanagh, S. L. (2017). Antigone's legacy: A feminist psychoanalytic of an Other sexual difference. *MAMSIE: Studies in the Maternal, 9*(1), 4. http://doi.org/10.16995/sim.223

Copjec, Joan. 2004. *Imagine There's No Woman: Ethics and Sublimation*. The MIT Press. https://doi.org/10.7551/mitpress/3668.001.0001.

Ettinger, Bracha. 1997. The Feminine/Prenatal Weaving in Matrixial Subjectivity-as-Encounter. *Psychoanalytic Dialogues* 7 (3): 367–405.

Ettinger, Bracha. 2000a. Art as the Transport-Station of Trauma. In *Bracha Lichtenberg Ettinger: Artworking, 1985–1999*. Ludion: Palais des Beaux-Arts.

Ettinger, Bracha Lichtenberg. 2000c. Transgressing With-In-To the Feminine. In *Differential Aesthetics: Art Practices, Philosophy and Feminist Understandings*, ed. Penny Florence and Nicola Foster, 1st ed. Routledge. https://doi.org/10.4324/9781315182735-13.

Ettinger, Bracha Lichtenberg. 2001. The Red Cow Effect: The Metramorphosis of Hallowing the Hollow and Hollowing the Hallow. In *He Said, She Says: An RSVP to the Male Text*, ed. Mica Howe and Sarah Appleton Aguiar. Fairleigh Dickinson University Press.

Ettinger, Bracha. 2006. *The Matrixial Borderspace*, Theory out of Bounds. Vol. 28. University of Minnesota Press.

Ettinger, Bracha Lichtenberg. 2007. Diotima and the Matrixial Transference: Psychoanalytical Encounter-Event as Pregnancy in Beauty. In *Beyond the Threshold: Explorations of Liminality in Literature*, ed. Hein Viljoen and N. Chris. Van der Merwe. Peter Lang.

Ettinger, Bracha Lichtenberg. 2009. Fragilization and Resistance. *Studies in the Maternal* 1 (2): 1–31. https://doi.org/10.16995/sim.141.

Ettinger, Bracha. 2010. Antigone With(out) Jocaste. In *Interrogating Antigone in Postmodern Philosophy and Criticism*, ed. Stephen Elliot Wilmer and Audrone Žukauskaitė. Oxford University Press.

Ettinger, Bracha Lichtenberg. 2016. Laius Complex and Shocks of Maternality: With Franz Kafka and Sylvia Plath. In *Interdisciplinary Handbook of Trauma and Culture*, ed. Haviva Pedaya, David Gurevitz, Yuval Neria, and Yochai Ataria. Springer International Publishing.

Freeland, Charles. 2013. *Antigone, in Her Unbearable Splendor: New Essays on Jacques Lacan's The Ethics of Psychoanalysis*. State University of New York Press.

Honig, Bonnie. 2011. Ismene's Forced Choice: Sacrifice and Sorority in Sophocles' Antigone. *Arethusa* 44 (1): 29–68.

Irigaray, Luce. 2010. The Eternal Irony of the Community. In *Feminist Readings of Antigone*, SUNY Series in Gender Theory, ed. Fanny Söderbäck. SUNY Press.

Kristeva, Julia. 2010. Limit and Horizon. In *Feminist Readings of Antigone*, ed. Fanny Söderbäck, 1st ed. State University of New York Press.

Lacan, Jacques. 1992. *The Ethics of Psychoanalysis 1959–1960: The Seminar of Jacques Lacan*. Edited by Jacques-Alain Miller. Translated by Dennis Porter. Book VII. W. W. Norton & Company Inc.

Lacan, Jacques. 2006g. The Subversion of the Subject and the Dialectic of Desire in the Freudian Unconscious. In *Écrits: The First Complete Edition in English*. Translated by Bruce Fink. W.W. Norton & Company.

Lacan, Jacques. 2006l. The Function and Field of Speech and Language in Psychoanalysis. In *Écrits: The First Complete Edition in English*. Translated by Bruce Fink. W.W. Norton & Company.
Lacan, Jacques. 2011. The Seminar of Jacques Lacan: Book X: Anxiety: 1962–1963. Unpublished manuscript. Translated by Cormac Gallagher.
Morel, Geneviève. 2018. *The Law of the Mother: An Essay on the Sexual Sinthome*. 1st ed. Routledge.
Sjöholm, Cecilia. 2004. *The Antigone Complex: Ethics and the Invention of Feminine Desire*. 1st ed. Stanford University Press.
Söderbäck, Fanny, ed. 2010. *Feminist Readings of Antigone*, SUNY Series in Gender Theory. SUNY Press.
Sophocles. 1984. *The Three Theban Plays: Antigone, Oedipus the King, Oedipus at Colonus*. Translated by Robert Fagles. Penguin Classics.

8

Conclusion: Ettinger and Lacan: A Sexual Impasse That Will Not Stop Being Written

Bracha Ettinger's psychoanalytic project is to acknowledge the vitally important role of the mother in psychoanalysis and to consider the Real, phantasmatic, and sub-Symbolic significance of reproduction. In this book, I emphasize the importance of reading Ettinger alongside Lacan. It should not be forgotten that Ettinger's matrixial theory is developed in relation to Lacanian concepts and theories of the subject. Her critical matrixial supplement to Lacanian psychoanalysis is motivated by a dissatisfaction with his interpretation of the Woman who does not exist, the signifier which does not include attention to procreation, and his representation of the m/Other as endangering the child through her overbearing desire and jouissance. As I have shown in previous chapters, Ettinger develops a theory of the matrixial whereby the Woman exists, she offers the *a-link* as a supplement to Lacan's *object a* (non-object cause of desire), develops a theory of severality (the subject as encounter), formulates the matrixial gaze as distinct from the phallic gaze, and builds upon Lacan's writings on Feminine jouissance and the m/Other. Ettinger's theory of the matrixial posits a Feminine axis of difference whereby the subject is not only constituted by the signifier (as in Lacan), but by a primary

S. L. Cavanagh, *Bracha L. Ettinger and Jacques Lacan*, The Palgrave Lacan Series,
https://doi.org/10.1007/978-3-032-23293-9_8

relation (or borderlinking) to the m/Other and, later, to others with whom they are trans-connected in the matrixial sub-Symbolic.

Without negating the originality and importance of Ettingerian psychoanalysis, it is necessary to understand how her foundational concepts relating to the matrixial correspond to Lacan's writings and clinical observations about the weaning (*sevrage*) complex,[1] the maternal imago and the interhuman. Lacan's references to the mother, the maternal realm, and the maternal object, however sparce, are inseparable from his theorization of the phallus, the Imaginary and the Symbolic (Barzilai 1999). But for Ettinger, these central concepts must be articulated from a non-phallic perspective. Not only does Ettinger offer a critique of Lacanian psychoanalysis, but also a Feminine supplement that makes important contributions to feminist theory and to post-Lacanian psychoanalytic thought.

In Lacan's writing, the mother lacks and the child becomes her phallic object. Ettinger is critical of Lacan's position relating to the necessity of the paternal metaphor (the Name of the Father), the way it is thought to introduce a necessary triangle, or third position, from which the child-toddler can take distance from the desire and jouissance of the m/Other. In Ettinger's view, the matrixial does not pose a danger to the child. It is, in my reading, entirely subjectivizing in Ettingerian thought (unless, of course, matrixial links are torn or severed). For Lacanians who believe in the importance of the significatory cut and the dangers of an overbearing maternal jouissance, questions arise about how we might theorize ambivalence, rivalrous identification and aggression in the maternal realm. Ettinger places aggression on the phallic side, but there is, nevertheless, a question about how the paternal metaphor might be relevant to the matrixial subject. Equally, questions need to be asked about the masculine in relation to the matrixial. Is, for example, the masculine necessarily phallic, and what function might it have in relation to the matrixial? For Ettinger, the Feminine dimension is relevant to everyone despite gender identity or sexual morphology, but the function of the masculine, in relation to the matrixial-Feminine, is in need of further exploration.

[1] See *Les complexes familiaux dans la formation de l'individu* (1938), volume 8 of the *Encyclopédie française*.

While some of Ettinger's writings posit Lacanian theory and matrixial theory as wholly distinct there are, as I argue, important areas of synergy and overlap. Each previous chapter demonstrates how Ettinger's theory relates to and departs from Lacan's writings, but I also foreground the ways Ettinger and Lacan are, in fact, theorizing the same phenomena relating to the subject and the m/Other. In my interpretation, Ettinger's formulation of the Other Sexual Difference (OSD) is not inconsistent with Lacan's notes on the Other, the unconscious (as trans-individual), and the Other jouissance. The Woman who does not exist for Lacan is also not unlike like the Ettingerian Woman who lacks inscription in the Symbolic, as I discuss in Chap. 4.

In this final chapter, I draw additional parallels and points of divergence in Ettinger and Lacan with respect to the Woman; childbirth and intrauterine experience; the m/Other; and the subject. In so doing, I highlight the importance and originality of Ettinger's approach without loosing site of the way it corresponds to Lacan's original teachings.

The Woman

While the Lacanian Woman does not exist in full under the phallic premise, the Ettingerian Woman exists in full in the matrixial. She is described as an assemblage of changing borderlines and linkages between partial-subjects in the Feminine-matrixial sub-Symbolic. Unlike the Lacanian Woman who experiences an Other jouissance, the Ettingerian Woman is bound by desire and jouissance in the borderlinking. The Woman is not an individual subject in Ettingerian theory, but a site of co-emergence, a border-Other.

Ettinger likens the Woman to a matrixial weave which calls to mind Lacanian knots and quilting points. But for Ettinger, the matrixial weave gives form to Woman as a transitive sex difference as explained in Chap. 4. She functions as an anchor for the OSD. This definition of the Woman enables Ettinger to theorize partial subjectivity involving sub-subjectivity and trans-subjectivity, as discussed in Chap. 2. This notion of partial subjectivity is distinct from the Lacanian definition of the subject. While the Lacanian subject of language is mediated by the desire and demand of the

Other, the Ettingerian subject is a condition of transitivity that touches upon a Feminine-Real.

What we might call the matrixial touch occurs in the matrixial sub-stratum (or sub-Symbolic). As outlined in Chaps. 2 and 3, the matrixial sub-stratum is neither Oedipal nor phallic. The matrixial sub-stratum is, for Ettinger, a dimension of Feminine experience grounded in the primary relation to the m/Other. In this dimension, borderlinkings co-occur between partial-subjects and Others (or *non-I*'s). They harken back to unremembered primary experiences in utero. As such, the borderlinkings are not known (exactly), but felt and sensed. The borderlinking is sexual but not about what Lacan would call a jouissance of the organ. Nor is it about *object a*. Rather, the borderlinking is, for Ettinger, an *a-link* or, in other words, a seduction into life. Thus, the borderlinking is essential to the matrixial subject-as-several.

There is, as both scholars would agree, a non-equivalence between the masculine and the Feminine, but for Ettinger, the Woman must be theorized (or apprehended) if not signified directly. I do not believe Lacan would disagree. In fact, he believes that the Woman is something other than what can be signified. Feminists might not like the way he, sometimes flippantly, says the Woman does not exist, but perhaps the origins of sexism exist, at least in part, in the way her excess is difficult to comprehend. Lacanian theory gives rise to a form of feminism concerned with the way the Woman is not-all because she exists, in part, outside language. Post-Lacanian feminists like Ettinger are interested not only in the m/Other and procreation but also in how the un-signifiable Feminine relates to subjectivity.

While both theorists define the Woman differently, there is a shared understanding that there is more to the subject of the Woman that can be said. Ettinger's formulation of the Other axis of sexual difference can also be read in relation to Lacan's theorization of the Other jouissance experienced, he says, by women alone—both are experiential domains, or fields, that are unbarred by the signifier. Although Ettinger claims that Lacan folds what she calls the matrixial into the phallic dimension, it is productive to ask if the phallic dimension can be, or is, entirely cut-off from the matrixial-Feminine dimension. If, as Ettinger contends, a man can access the Feminine-matrixial, he is not entirely cut off from the

Feminine dimension (2000). Moreover, the Feminine, as Ettinger explains, does not disappear in the life of the subject, even as it defies direct representation in phallic terms.

As I have argued in my previous work on Tiresias as applied to transgender studies (Cavanagh 2016, 2018, 2019, 2022), Ettinger's article on the Transgression-within-to-the-Feminine (2000), as it relates to the case of the blind prophet who changes sex, illustrates that the man has to know something of the Feminine dimension. For Ettinger, the Feminine dimension is occluded in Lacan's sexuation graph and this is a problem from the perspective of the matrixial.

Lacan may, in fact, agree. For both theorists, there is more to the subject than can be signified and sexuality is not reducible to sexuation (masculine or feminine positions). Indeed, Lacan never tires of commenting upon the way subjects do not neatly fit into his formulation of sexual positioning. He says, for example, that hysterics do not become women (or men) (Cavanagh 2019), that mothers cannot easily be placed on the feminine side,[2] and that because feminine jouissance has nothing to do with the man as *object a* (cause of desire) it is unrelated to the masculine side (and thus unrepresentable). It follows that the Feminine field of sexual difference exists for both Ettinger and Lacan. The difference is in the way each approaches what cannot be said about the Feminine. Ettinger, as we have already seen, develops an elaborate theory of the matrixial borderspace whereas, I argue, Lacan approaches the Feminine dimension through his writings on the Other.

The best example is to be found in Lacan's writings on Antigone in *Seminar VII* as I discuss in the previous chapter. He refers to two dimensions (or fields) relating to the subject, one of which is beyond the reach of signification. Lacan's analysis pivots around what he calls Antigone's *Até*, a limit concerning the field of the Other (1992, 277). The *Até* refers to a Greek Goddess who acts upon a deadly and brash violence. Although

[2] It is interesting to note that Lacan had trouble positioning the one who occupies the maternal position on the right side of the sexuation graph. As Giovanna di Giovanni argues, maternity is about 'having' a child (phallus), not 'being' (a phallus), which is a masculine solution (referenced in Adrian Price, 2008, 57). Price (2008) further explains that the "mother has, and the woman has not and makes something of this lack" (61). Mothers can thus not be all 'woman' in the Lacanian sense.

the matrixial field is not deadly, but futuristic and life-giving, both the matrixial and the Feminine *Até* in Lacan are what ultimately matter to Antigone. Antigone's beauty radiates from what Lacan calls an intermediary between two fields that can be differentiated (248). Her beauty involves a blinding spectre, something that resides at a limit where a metamorphosis may occur. This metamorphic possibility, which Lacan links back to the writings of Ovid (265), are contiguous with Ettinger's theory of *metra*morphosis in the matrixial borderlinking (described in Chap. 3). Equally, Antigone is, for Lacan, driven by a force beyond the King and the field of the signifier where the rule of law can be inscribed. This field that resides at the limit for Lacan is, in my interpretation, an entry point to the Ettingerian matrixial.

Although Lacan is more likely to refer to previous generations than to the m/Other, both theorists know that there is something relating to Jocasta that drives Antigone. While Jocasta goes largely unnamed in Lacan's writings on the Sophocles heroine, he does say that the m/Other's desire is fundamental to the structure—to the structure of the drama, and to the structure of our lives. In my view, there is something of unique importance about the m/Other that Ettinger approaches in ways that Lacan does not. Who the m/Other is to the girl-daughter becoming (or not-becoming) a woman is under theorized in Lacan and in psychoanalysis more broadly. By centering procreation and the m/Other, Ettinger offers new insight into the case study of Dora, Lol Stein in the Marguerite Duras novel, and to Antigone of the Oedipal trilogy. Each has symptom-struggles involving the m/Other. While Lacan gestures to elements of the daughter's experience vis-a-vis the m/Other, Ettinger develops an extensive vocabulary inclusive of mother–daughter complexes involving the OSD.

As discussed in previous chapters, the OSD is set in motion by a primordial relation to the m/Other and this is, in my assessment, the most original and important element of Ettinger's theory of the matrixial. From the perspective of the OSD, the Woman is a site of co-emergence involving partial subjects, the self and the Other. This involves another kind of relation to the Other, one that recalls a primary jouissance alongside the corpo-Reality of the mother. In the case study of Dora, the story of Lol Stein, and the drama of Antigone, Ettinger articulates the significance of the m/Other and the OSD to the girl-daughter.

Childbirth and Intrauterine

As discussed in Chap. 2, Ettinger contends that Freudian and Lacanian theories neglect pre-birth phenomenon and the OSD involving the m/Other. Her claim is that childbirth is unthought and largely omitted in psychoanalytic theory because it is, for the boy-child, dangerous and injurious to his narcissism as Freud reasoned (see Chap. 3). While Ettinger may be correct in her assessment of Freud and in her claim that Lacan forecloses on the womb as a subjective space of difference, there are poignant however occasional references to the womb in Lacan's writings that nuance her claim. For instance, Lacan does, albeit sparingly, refer to procreation and to mothering in his teachings. He saw pregnancy fantasies as being relevant to at least one clinical case involving a male patient (2006o 456). While discussing the writings of German psychiatrist Ida Macalpine (1889–1974), Lacan sympathizes with her wish to theorize procreation fantasies (456). Not unlike Ettinger, Macalpine felt, according to Lacan, the "need to tie this [procreation] fantasy to a symbolic structure" (456) in relation to the transference. In *The Psychoanalytic Act: Seminar XV*, Lacan writes that birth is authentically recognized when it is forgotten, when it is mis-recognized (2002 [1967–1968], 152). This is not a sexist remark for Lacan, but an acknowledgment of something vital relating to the maternal-Feminine that cannot be remembered or recognized as such. Like Eurydice[3] who, in Ettinger's interpretation, exists when she is unseen by Orpheus in the Greek myth (and appears in Ettinger's paintings), the experience of birth does not lend itself to Imaginary capture or to Symbolic representation. It is unremembered and unarticulated: lost but nevertheless present.

Thus, it should not be surprising that Ettinger and Lacan both refer to hauntings. For Lacan, we are haunted by images of castration,

[3]For a discussion of Eurydice in Ettingerian art See: (Buci-Glucksmann 1999; and Kisiel 2019, 2020).

emasculation, mutilation, dismemberment, dislocation, evisceration, devouring, and bursting open of the body. Ettinger interprets hauntings as involving the ghost-like figure of the m/Other or, in her artworks, Eurydice and Persephone.[4] While Ettinger's focus on the m/Other directs attention to the scene of birth and to the corpo-Real specificity of the maternal body, Lacan's haunting have a more oblique relation to the m/Other. For Lacan, castration is not about the loss of a penis-organ (or any specific body part); it is a more generalized fear of subjective fragmentation and loss of identity. Fear of castration is often experienced in relation to the m/Other because it harkens back to an un-cognized scene of birth. What goes unremembered is both alienating and germane to the subject. For Ettinger, this forgotten past-scene of birth is not entirely forgotten, but felt and intuited at the level of the matrixial.

While Lacan did not theorize a Feminine axis of difference to supplement the Symbolic register in his typology of the human subject, he knows that the maternal instinct can not be understood through phallic mediation. In, for example, his presentation titled "Guiding Remarks for a Convention on Female Sexuality," Lacan questions whether "phallic mediation accounts for everything drive-related that can manifest itself in women, especially the whole current of maternal instinct" (2006e, 614). While he does not theorize the maternal instinct, he acknowledges that the whole of human experience is not reducible to the phallic dimension. He equates the pre-verbal with the preconscious and agrees that it is central to the subject's "intraworldly *Gestalt*" (1997, 164).

Having said this, it must also be acknowledged that Lacan wrote, in his early work, that there is "no such thing as a prediscursive reality. Every reality is founded and defined by a discourse" (1999, 32). Despite this proclamation, Lacan spends considerable time on the question of the preverbal in *Seminar III* (on psychosis) and concludes that this "pre- or even extraverbal communication is always present in analysis is not in doubt, but it is a question of seeing what it is that constitutes the properly analytic field" (1997, 164). For Lacan, the proper focus of clinical work is

[4] The image on the book-cover is titled Eurydice – Persephone, 2021. The art-work is India ink and aquarelle on paper. The painting has been exhibited at the Fondazione Antonio Dalle Nogare in Bolzano, Italy; High Art Gallery in Paris, France; and K21 Kunstsammlung Nordrhein-Westfalen, Düsseldorf, Germany.

the subject's discourse because it is upon the subject's unconscious—structured as it is, like a language—that the psychoanalytic method is based. In his writing on Feminine sexuality, Lacan contends without equivocation that just because "everything that is analyzable is sexual does not mean that everything that is sexual is accessible to analysis" (2006e, 614).

Both Lacan and Ettinger agree that the pre-verbal operations of psychical life involve different pathways of communication to those of the verbal. As shown in previous chapters, Ettinger theorizes elements of human experience beginning with conception that are unrelated to the signifier. Additionally, she regards these matrixial elements of experience, tied to the m/Other, as worthy of psychoanalytic and clinical attention. A careful reading of Lacan suggests that he may, in fact, agree. While he believes, like Ettinger, that procreation escapes the Symbolic, he seems to believe that there is something else relating to procreation that is covered over by the symbolic tapestry. Lacan writes:

> There is nevertheless one thing that evades the symbolic tapestry, it's procreation in its essential root – that one being is born from another. In the symbolic order procreation is covered by the order instituted by this succession between beings. But nothing in the symbolic explains the fact of their individuation, the fact that beings come from beings. The entire symbolism declares that creatures don't engender creatures, that a creature is unthinkable without a fundamental creation. In the symbolic nothing explains creation. (1997, 179)

In this passage, Lacan clearly acknowledges the mysteries of creation along with the way procreation escapes the Symbolic tapestry. He also refers to an affective co-relation between subjects in the procreative encounter that Ettinger's theory of the matrixial borderspace pinpoints more directly. Ettinger's psychoanalysis gives form to un-cognized memories of the early mother-to-be/late fetal sexual relation that leaves trace inscriptions, mediate affects, and produces internal sensations that operate in what she calls the sub-Symbolic (or matrixial substratum).

The m/Other

Ettinger contends that Lacan neglects procreation and the m/Other in his teachings. As I have shown in Chap. 5, Lacan says very little about the m/Other in the case study of Dora. He says nothing about the m/Other in his homage to Marguerite Duras and in his discussion of the fictive-character Lol Stein. Lacan also does not theorize the vital role of Jocasta in *Antigone*, the m/Other who is, as he says elsewhere, foundational to the structure. It must also be acknowledged that there are more references to the paternal function than to the maternal function in Lacan's teachings.

In my view, there is an interesting contradiction at play in Lacanian psychoanalysis vis-a-vis the m/Other. On the one hand, there is, as has already been stated, a neglect of the mother in his discourse. It is unfortunate that Lacan does not say more about the mother given that she is, in his own theorizing, the "terminal point, the abolition of the whole world of demand" (1992, p. 68) for the man. For him, the m/Other is also related to the drives and the Real (the register beyond signification). He refers to the almightiness of the mother (2020, 185–186) and to the mother as that which "structures [the] man's unconscious" (1992, 68). The mother is also, for Lacan, the unconscious focal point of courtly love as he proclaims in *Seminar VII*. His analysis of courtly love, as one example, reveals that the *Thing* of relevance to desire is the Feminine *Thing* metonymically linked to the mother (or primary Other) (Cavanagh 2022).

Although Ettinger accuses Lacan of reducing the m/Other to the *Thing* (*das Ding*), he is not so reductive as that. For example, in *Seminar VII* Lacan characterizes the mother not exactly as the maternal *Thing* (*das Ding*), but as occupying the "place of that thing, of a *das Ding*" (1992, 67). *Das Ding* is a lost object that was never there in the first place, something that covers over a lack in being (58).

In Lacanian terms, what lacks (and acts as a catalyst of desire) is not the mother, but something that exceeds articulation and representation. By this, I take Lacan to mean that there is something more to the subject and to being that not only concerns the Real event of procreation, but to what Ettinger calls the matrixial. Before the mirror-stage, the toddler experiences fragmentation, a lack of distinction between the mother's body and itself. Elsewhere, Lacan says that we are, in this stage, *hommelettes* (scrambled) (1997 [1963–1964], 197). What we might call this zone of non-distinction is not unlike the matrixial where the *I* and the *non-I* are borderlinked in matrixial terms. Where differences lie, as I will explain below, is with respect to how Ettinger develops a theory of severality distinct from the Lacanian *hommelette* (see Chap. 2).

I will return to the question of the Ettingerian subject in what follows, but here suffice to say that Lacan does not underestimate the importance of the mother. In *Seminar IV*, Lacan insists that his students understand the power of the mother, the way imaginary objects are bound to the maternal body, and the way the "mother constitutes a virtual field of symbolic annihilation, from which each of the objects to come will in turn draw their symbolic value" (2020, 178). But how then do we explain the relative lack of theorizing relevant to the maternal function compared to the paternal function (or Name of the Father)? From a purely quantitative account, the mother does not appear as regularly as does the father and is not theorized as rigorously as she should be in Lacan's teachings given his own statements about her grandiosity in the life of the subject.

I contend that it is not (only) that Lacan neglects the mother in his theorizing, but that the mother has been incorporated into his theorization of the Other. Consider that for Lacan, the Other's discourse is the unconscious. In his discussion of desire in the psychoanalytic treatment, Lacan notes that the "subject's own speech is a message to him, first of all, because it is produced in the Other's locus. It originates in that locus and is worded as such not only because his demand is submitted to the Other's code, but because his demand is dated by this Other's locus (and even time)" (2006k, 529). At the same time, in *Seminar V*, Lacan refers to the mother as providing "the sign of signifying articulation" for the child.

He seems to be using the mother and the Other interchangeably or, at least, establishing a metonym between the two. In a brief mention of D.W. Winnicott, Lacan refers to the "function of mothering in the genesis of the object" (511). But Lacan also contends that desire testifies to the impossibility of liberating oneself from the discourse of the Other, of speaking in a way that would incarnate a desire (and discourse) separable from the Other, thereby alleviating a split internal to the subject which is indicated by what Lacan calls the "slanted bar of noble bastardy" (Ecrits, 530). The metonymic slide from mother to Other is evident in his discourse. From the masculine point of view, Lacan tells us that the Other's desire [*le désir de l'Autre*] is about what the mother wants, the phallus (2006e, 617). Who the mother is from what we might call a Feminine non-point of view (recall the off-centre matrixial gaze discussed in Chaps. 3 and 4) is undertheorized.

But Lacan does approach the m/Other's desire from another angle. He returns to Freud's discussion of the *Fort Da* game. Contra Freud, Lacan reasons that it is not the mother's absence, but her presence, that the child (Freud's nephew) is attempting to master. In *Seminar X*, Lacan refers to the maternal womb as engendering anxiety which he defines as a lack of lack. When there is a "lack of lack", and the "mother is always on his back", the child experiences anxiety. Lacan contends that where the m/Other lacks the subject hears a demand to be something in and for the mother. Her desire (as demand) provokes anxiety, anxiety which Lacan says "we wish she would tone down" (2006g, 698), and one that must be mitigated by a father (or a substitute) whose job it is to "unite…desire to the Law" (698).

Despite what Ettinger may, quite rightly, view as a sexist reference to the mother being on a boy-child's metaphorical back, Lacan is meaning to underscore the influence of the m/Other's desire and jouissance (which I will discuss below) on the child-subject. Lacan credits the Name-of-the-Father, or the paternal function, for saving the male-subject from the mother. The father ensures that the "man does not remain bound [attaché] to the sexual service of his mother…[and] that the Law institutes…the prohibition of incest" (2006p, 723).[5]

For Ettinger, there is a problem with the way the borderlinking between mother and child-toddler-fetus (which dates back to unremembered time in utero) is interpreted, by Lacan, as parasitic. Indeed, Lacan refers to the embryo-fetus-newborn as existing in a "parasitical relation to the mother's body, the breast appears as the same kind of organ---to be understood

[5] While some Lacanian analysts would claim that the desire of the m/Other can (and does) overwhelm the subject and that part of analytic work is about a relinquishing of the Other's desire, comparable worries about the desire of the Father are significantly less pronounced in the literature.

as the ectopia of one individual onto another—as that constituted by the placenta at the beginning of the growth of a certain type of organism which remains specified by this intersection" (2006f, 719). The intersection of concern to Lacan is Real and without subjective or Symbolic demarcation. This is what makes it parasitical. For Ettinger, this intersection is the borderlinking foundational to the matrixial-Feminine. She thus challenges the Lacanian representation of the relationship between the embryo-fetus-child and the becoming-mother as parasitic or fused.

While Lacan may be concerned about the after-birth effects of what he views as a lack of subjective demarcation in utero, the m/Other is consistently described in his teachings as posing a threat to the child. For Lacan, the desire of the m/Other is dangerously jouissant. Her desire is not experienced by the infant-child as nurturing so much as it is experienced as a threat. Lacan portrays a child in fear of being swallowed up or eaten-alive by the m/Other in his example of the praying mantis or the crocodile mother. In an early paper on aggressiveness in psychoanalysis presented in Brussels in 1948, Lacan refers in passing to the aggressions of a mother toward her homosexual son and says that "her permanent aggressiveness as a virile woman had taken its toll" (2006a, 84). It is difficult to read this passage without interpreting it as both sexist and homophobic which, in fact, it may be. But the critical point to make is that Lacan does not suggest that the aggression of the mother causes homosexuality in men. He is critical of determinist formulations when it comes to sexual object choice. The Lacanian objective here, as I understand it, is to explicate the way the phantasies of the mother are passed on to the child (2006q, 632). But more than this, he contends that our desire is the Other's desire because it is formulated in relation to what the Other desires; the first Other, again, being the mother. This is of great consequence to psychoanalysis because the "subject here makes himself the instrument of the Other's jouissance" (2006g, 697).

Ettinger astutely observes that Lacan's occasional discussions of maternal jouissance and pregnancy tend to occur in close proximity to his writings on psychosis. For example, his writings, quoted above, on procreation are taken from Book III, his seminar on *The Psychosis*, 1955–1956. From Ettinger's perspective, reproductive phenomenon that are beyond signification turn into "residue, refuse, empty bodies" (1997, 259) in Lacan's writings. He also refers to the delusion of procreation as it effected the symptomatology of Daniel Paul Schreber, a German supreme court-judge, who wrote eloquently about his experience of psychosis, and associated feelings of becoming a Woman, in *Memoirs of My Nervous Illness* (2000) (original German title *Denkwürdigkeiten eines Nervenkranken*).

Specifically, Lacan observes that Schreber's first attack occurs when he identifies with the mother's desire. Schreber assumes "his mother's desire, triggers, as a result of being shaken up, the dissolution of the imaginary tripod (note that it was in his mother's apartment, where he had taken refuge, that the subject had his first attack of anxious confusion with suicidal raptus…)" (2006o, 472). It can be difficult to parse out the moments when Lacanian discourse is sexist and when he is explicating something, relating to the m/Other, that is psychoanalytically significant. Ettinger is right to draw our attention to the sexist construction of the m/Other in Lacanian discourse, the way it is informed by his thinking about psychosis, etc. But, at the same time, we must consider the fact that Lacan might not be intending to blame the mother so much as he is intending to describe the dangers of maternal jouissance when it exists, for the child, without interdiction; that is, without an intervening signifier or paternal metaphor. Let us also remember that in Lacan's interpretation, Schreber did not have an operative signifier for procreation. This is what, in Lacan's considered view, inaugurates the original crisis. While there is always something in excess of the signifier, the psychotic experiences a return of that which escapes symbolization from without as a verbal hallucination. If, for example, there is no signifier for "woman" or "procreation," it returns from outside the subject and is experienced as persecutory because it is unbarred (or unnamed). This is not to say that actual women or mothers, or even phantasies of procreation, cause psychotic breaks but that there is a significatory foreclosure in the psychotic subject that is a problem of language. Lacan writes that "whatever is refused in the symbolic order, in the sense of *Verwerfung*, reappears in the real" (1997, 13).

In his discussion of Schreber, Lacan does refer to a pre-discursive phenomenon before the "coming into play of the divine discourse…[of] what could be called a trans-space linked to the structure of the signifier and of meaning, a spatialization prior to any possible dualization of the phenomenon of language" (141). Read in Ettingerian terms, it is possible that this trans-space is akin to her formulation of the trans-subjective discussed in Chap. 3. But for Ettinger, this trans-space would not be understood as infantile or psychotic but as central to the OSD. The trans-subjective in Ettinger may, in fact, be eluded to in Lacan's reference to the "*infans* state." In a lecture Lacan gave at the French Philosophical Society in 1957, he says that "we are...born a second time, in leaving behind the state which is rightly known as the *infans* state, for it is without speech --- namely, the symbolic order constituted by language, and the moment of the concrete universal discourse and of all the furrows opened up by it at this time, in which we had to find lodging" (2006i, 371). In effect, the Lacanian subject is born twice: once in the *infans* state and again in language—the latter involving alienation by the signifier.

Ettinger theorizes what Lacan refers to as the "*infans* state" without speech, but she does so without reducing it to a parasitical relationship. For Ettinger, matrixial subjectivity involves an enlarged subjectivity inclusive of Others (*non-I*'s) in matrixial alliance, as discussed in Chap. 3. What she also calls severality (the subject-as-encounter) begins in utero and is central to the OSD.

The Ettingerian Subject, the Feminine, and the Woman

In a Forward to *The Matrixial Borderspace* (Ettinger 2006d), Judith Butler writes that Ettinger is "asking us to reformulate the very relation between the subject and its other, and to ask what precedes this encounter in which the phallus seeks to confirm its status, where the feminine acts only as a faulty mirror in the circuitry of that [phallic] narcissism" (Butler 2006, x). Griselda Pollock's introduction to the same edited collection further explains that Ettingerian psychoanalysis "invites us to consider human subjectivity beyond the effects of Oedipal, pre-Oedipal and even anti-Oedipal mechanisms, as well as beyond intersubjective object relations...[matrixial] subjectivity operates as a shifting perspective, as *encounter*" (2006, 14).

As discussed in Chap. 2, Ettinger defines the matrix as an "unconscious space of simultaneous emergence and fading of the *I* and the unknown non-I which is neither fused or rejected" (1996, 125). The first corporeal-psychic connection between *I* and *non-I* occurs inside the maternal womb where every *I* is tethered to female invisible corporeality and is a borderlinking to the m/Other's psychic environment (Ettinger 2006a, 70). The subject-encounter-event between the *I* and the *non-I* occurs in a shared borderspace on the outer reaches of a given matrixial web. It is a catalyst for Feminine desire (not to be confused with femininity or the Other jouissance). Desire in the borderlinking is not about amalgamation but co-emergent heterogeneity. Matrixial subjectivity is about differentiation, not fusion or symbiosis.[6] The matrixial is also not about cognition, but affects, non-conscious memory, and aesthetics. It is about "non-unifiable and linked space of a primary psychic relation the feminine" (Butler 2004, 98).

Building upon Lacan's conceptualization of the Other jouissance and Lévinas's later work on the Feminine, Ettinger gives form to a notion of the Feminine that is un-cut by the signifier as discussed in Chap. 4. The matrixial is about Feminine difference, alterity, and (non-phallic) difference. Ettinger explains that the matrix is a "feminine dimension of plurality and difference of the several in joint subjectivity" (Ettinger 1996, 152). From Ettinger's perspective, the Feminine dimension of experience is eclipsed in/by the language of the phallus germane to Lacanian teachings. For her, the matrixial Feminine is about the inter-human. But it resonates with the Lacanian unconscious which he defines, in part, as trans-individual. A difference lies in how each theorist articulates the Other and otherness as related to subjectivity. For Lacan, desire is the desire of the Other, but for Ettinger, Feminine desire involves borderlinking to and with the m/Other. Unlike Lacan who regards the Feminine as a radical Other, Ettinger focuses on the matrixial borderlinking between

[6] In a radical departure from psychoanalytic theorists like, for example, Christopher Bollas, who understands the late intrauterine encounter in terms of symbiosis and "psychosomatic sensations of *fusion*" (2006, 78), Ettinger argues that this encounter is subjectivizing and not predicated upon symbiosis or fusion. She claims that this encounter is predicated upon an Other Feminine sexual difference that is subjectivizing (and that can be signified in a wider symbolic). Furthermore, it is, for Ettinger, crucial to the engendering of the "Self-with-other psychic dimension of subjectivity" (2006d, 82).

the subject and the Other as intimate and apprehendable. For her, the Feminine is not a radical Other, but a pre-discursive dimension central to an enlarged subjectivity: a "shareable dimension of subjectivity" where both *I* and *non-I* "co-emerge and co-inhabit a joint space" (Ettinger 2006d, 65).

This formation of subjectivity adds complexity to the Lacanian definition of the subject constituted by the signifier. But while matrixial subjectivity is, for Ettinger, separate from phallic subjectivity (mediated by the signifier), I question the extent to which matrixial elements of the subject are absent in Lacan's theory of subjectivity. For example, we might consider how severality, in the Feminine-matrixial, is related to what Lacan calls the "unassimilable intersubjective" (1992, 17). I would also suggest that Ettinger's notion of the trans-subjective is not too far removed from Lacan's writing on the impossibility of the two in the ternary articulation. "Between two, whatever they may be, there is always the One and the Other, the One and the *a*, and the Other cannot in any way be taken as a One" (Lacan 1999, 49). Elsewhere, Lacan claims that there is One but that this One is not simple. The Lacanian subject is bound to the Other's desire and discourse, subject to the Other's demand and the unconscious demonstrates that this subject is split. While Ettinger contends that this split is also a link (*link-a*), and I would agree, it cannot be said that the Lacanian subject is (only) One. In fact, Lacan's writings on the Other in the One resonates with Ettinger's notion of the subject-as-encounter.

Indeed, both scholars agree that the subject cannot be without the Other. Although Ettinger distinguishes between the matrixial and the Lacanian Symbolic, the borderlinking (*a-link*) and the cut of language (*object a*), there are important areas of overlap that get lost when Ettingerian psychoanalysis is not read alongside Lacan's original teachings. From a Lacanian perspective, Ettinger elaborates upon the pre-object of jouissance foundational to Lacan's formulation of *object a*. Her scholarship also gives us a way to contemplate elements of experience relating to gestation and birth that are unremembered, yet vital to embodiment, affect, aesthetics and to what Lacan calls the Imaginary. From a feminist psychoanalytic perspective, Ettinger gives us a way to say more about the Woman who does not exist in Lacanian psychoanalysis.

As already noted, Ettinger offers her theory of the matrixial borderspace as a critical supplement to Lacan. But she also writes, on occasion, as though her formulation of the matrixial is entirely distinct from Lacan. In my view, it is a mistake to presume the latter when important components of her theory build upon Lacanian insights relating to Feminine sexuality and the m/Other. But this is not to say that there are not original and important insights in Ettingerian theory uniquely relevant to what cannot be said about the daughter's relation to the mother. As feminists have shown, psychoanalysis has not only been sexist but primarily focused on the conundrums of the male-son in Freud's writings on the Oedipal complex and in the Lacanian corpus (Grosz 2002; Moi 2004). Ettinger is correct to note occlusions in the Lacanian cannon relevant to the female-daughter, the maternal body, and to what Lacan refers to as "annulled objects" (2020, 179) with symbolic value appearing as, or under signifiers of, nothingness.

As I illustrate in the previous three chapters on Dora, Lol Stein, and Antigone, Lacan neglects the vital role of the m/Other in his theorizing while, paradoxically, acknowledging her centrality. For Lacan who writes in *Seminar VII* about "*das Ding*…[associated with the] mother, [and] also the object of incest…a forbidden good, and that there is no other good" (Lacan 1992, 70), it is shocking that he does not say more about Jocasta in relation to Antigone, about the absent mother in the case study of Dora, and the wail of the mother in the story of Lol Stein.

The Other Sexual Difference

Feminist readers of Lacan, Ettinger being one such reader, have elaborated upon the place of the Woman (Copjec 2004, 2015; Mitchell and Rose 1983; Ragland-Sullivan 2012, 2014; Rose 2005; Soler 2002, 2006; and Zupančič 2017) and the m/Other (Barzilai 1999; Smart 2021; and Tsolas 2022) in Lacan's teachings. But Ettinger may be the first to have formulated an OSD as discussed in Chap. 2. The OSD is predicated upon non-conscious and unconscious relations to the corpo-Real specificity of the birth-giving m/Other. Boys and girls alike must first negotiate Feminine sexual difference before Oedipal sexual difference becomes a question and sexual positions relating to the desire of the Other and jouissance can be established. In other words, the question of sexual difference for both the boy and girl is initially directed to the m/Other (or primary Other who may not be female).

But this does not make the situations of the girl-daughter's and the boy-son's relation to the m/Other the same. For Ettinger, like Lacan, it is important to acknowledge a domain of non-equivalence between the sexes (2001, 67). Equally, Ettinger focuses on the unique experiences of the birth-giving mother who is, in her words, always female. Even when the maternal post-natal figure is male, pregnancy always involves what she calls female reproductive capacity. This is not to say that the person giving birth may not be transmasculine or that they identify as female (or feminine), but that there must be a word to designate the corpo-Real specificity of the birth-giving mother/subject's body. As we have seen in the previous chapters, sexual morphology matters in the Ettingerian paradigm, as does reproductive capacity. But both are mediated by what Lacan calls the Real and the Imaginary which adds complexity to what would otherwise be essentialist (or binary) formulations of male-man and female-woman-potential-mother.

While more work needs to be done on what it means for a boy-son to differentiate from the m/Other and, equally, how he differentiates from the father or masculine position[7] (if, in fact, he does), Ettinger's focus is on the girl-daughter's relation to the m/Other. This is because the m/Other matters differently to the girl-daughter and also because the mother-daughter relation, or borderlinking, has often been occluded in psychoanalysis. For Ettinger, the girl-daughter has unique access to the matrixial sphere due to her reproductive capacity, imagined and Real. As I discuss in Chaps. 3 and 4, Ettinger regards the female-girl-daughter's relation to the matrixial as distinct from the male-boy-son's relation to the matrixial. She explains:

[7] See Ettinger's writing on the Laius Complex involving the son where she notes that the boy-son has his own unique conundrum to work out: that is his difference from another male (as father), what Ettinger calls the "the feminine man-to-man difference" (Ettinger, 2010, 10). Freud wrote much about the male-boy-son and his father under the auspices of the Oedipus complex. But, in Ettinger's formulation, the Father-son relation needs to be worked out from the perspective of a non-Oedipal Feminine difference.

> Female subjects have double access to the matrixial sphere in the Real because they experience the womb both as an archaic out-site and past-side—out of chronological time as "anterior" (this is true for males as well)—and as an in-side and future-side—as an actual, future, and "posterior" time (whether they are mothers or not). (2006d, 143)

The girl's exploration of Feminine-sexual difference is prompted by a "dawning and vanishing link with a m/Other in resonance with the I" (Ettinger 2010, 10). While Lacan agrees that the I is always in the domain of the Other, he does not, in Ettinger's assessment, make room in his theorizing for a primary jouissance specific to the mother-daughter resonance field. Ettinger elaborates:

> Sexual difference for the girl indexes another woman who holds the site – time-and-space—of the m/Other and of the Woman-beneath-the-Mother who is forever enveloped inside the archaic m/Other who, as a *non-I*, dwells in resonance with the I (daughter) within a relational field of encounter thought of, to begin with, not in terms of inter-subjective relationships or object-relation but of pregnant coexistence. (9)

As discussed in previous chapters, Ettinger interprets this relational resonance field in terms of matrixial incest (to be distinguished from sexual abuse which occurs after-birth).

Her writing on matrixial incest complicates our understanding of the incest taboo relevant to Freud and Lacan. The Ettingerian formulation of the pre-birth incestuous liaison is a case in point. For Ettinger, the first sexual difference is with-in and between the *I* and the m/Other (as first *non-I*). But this is not altogether different from Lacan's interpretation of what occurs between neighbouring generations. While there may be no sexual relation between men and women (as sexuated subjects), there is, for Lacan, something like a sexual relation between neighbouring generations that the incest prohibition wards off. Specifically, Lacan says that there is "not sexual rapport except for neighbouring generations; namely, parents on the one hand, and children on the other. That's what the interdiction of incest wards off" (Lacan 1978,[8] quoted in Ettinger 1997, 389).

[8] Lacan, 1978. "Le moment de conclure" Unpublished manuscript (in Ettinger 1997, 405).

In *Seminar XXIII*, Lacan also concedes that something between the sexes works out from the perspective of the symptom. In the later Lacan, Ettinger finds a vital point of contact with the Lacanian corpus whereby she can theorize the non-prohibited incestuous encounter-event of birth and, by extension, the OSD where there is, in her analytic, a sexual rapport.

But the matrixial rapport is, for Ettinger, without aggression. It is Erotic, futuristic, and subjectifying. While there can be trauma in the borderlinking, Ettinger's writing on the matrixial does not make room for thought about the aggression of the m/Other. There can be severed and devastated matrixial links (as we have seen in her analysis of Dora, Lol Stein and Antigone), but the contempt and hate a mother may feel toward her daughter is not accounted for.[9] Because the mother is often blamed for child traumas in the psychoanalytic literature (Hirsch 1989), it is not surprising that feminist psychoanalytic theorists, like Ettinger, have been reluctant to theorize misogyny in the mother-daughter relation (or borderlinking) given the cultural tendency to blame the mother (Caplan 2002). But as a result, it is difficult to theorize what Caitlin Janzen (2022) refers to as a feminine death drive in Ettingerian scholarship.

Lacan, by contrast, does not hesitate to comment on the aggression of the m/Other. He says that she can be terrifying and devouring. For Lacan, the m/Other is not only associated with the primordial *Thing* around which desire orbits, but her desire can be overbearing. In Geneviève Morel's (2019) discussion about the "Law of the Mother" in Lacanian theory, she stresses how the child is subjugated to the mother's desire, to her law, to her discourse (*lalangue*), and is imprinted by this early object relation in symptomatic ways (2018, 306). The jouissance of the mother can be, for the child, beyond limits: hence the importance of the paternal function which triangulates the desire of the mother.

Ettinger does not dispute the influence of the mother's desire and jouissance upon the child. But she does not regard the mother as endangering the subjectivity of the child. Nor does she focus on what Melanie Klein would call hate, envy or rivalrous identification in the

[9] Nor is what Vaia Tsolas (2022) calls misogyny in mother-daughter relations theorized in Ettinger's writings.

mother-daughter object relation. I imagine that Ettinger would respond by underscoring the fact that matrixial theory is about severality and non-conscious relations to Others (as *non-I's*), not object relations. Thus, her theory of the matrixial does not involve object relations between individuals theorized by psychoanalysts like Klein and Donald Winnicott. Ettinger focuses on non-conscious affects, aesthetics, and trace-connections to the m/Other which are not reducible to identifiable actions on the part of individual subjects. The matrixial sphere involves, as mentioned above, borderlinkings between partial-subjects who share "phantasmatic and traumatic links" (Ettinger 2006a, 78), not the inter-subjective sphere where we act upon one another as individuals subject to the law.

Lacan would not dispute these co-effecting ties, but he would approach them from another angle. Indeed, as discussed in the previous chapter, Lacan focuses on Antigone and her death-bound devotion to her brother, Polynices. What Ettinger refers to as a matrixial borderlinking is, for Lacan, articulated through his conception of *object a* (*das Ding*), the *Ate*, and through his analytic of the Other which is, again, in the first instance the mother. While Ettinger's conceptualization of the Jocasta Complex is not, in my reading, at odds with Lacan's formulation of the m/Other, it gives us another way to consider what cannot be said or seen about the mother and daughter in the borderlinking inclusive of the jouissance relating to it.

More needs to be written about what Ettinger calls a primary sexual difference involving the m/Other. Lacanian teachings need to be augmented by feminist psychoanalytic theories of the maternal authored from the perspective of the girl-daughter so that we may better understand other axis of sexual difference. Equally, the over-emphasis upon sexual object choice (which Freud critiqued in *The Three Essays on the Theory of Sexuality* 2017 [1905]) and Lacanian sexual positioning, without attention to the maternal realm, obscures the Feminine dimension and what may be non-phallic sexualities. What bothers and excites us about sexuality, what feels compelling and devastating in equal measures, cannot be seen or said. This, Ettinger and Lacan agree upon. Let us also remember that Lacan mocks the discourse of sexual object choice. He says we are all *nullisexual*, troubled by the lack in the sexual couple. But where the m/Other figures in his theory of sexuality is not entirely clear.

In my view, there is an irreconcilable difference, what Lacan would call a sexual impasse. As I have argued throughout this book, Ettinger's theory of the matrixial cannot be subsumed into Lacan's writings on Feminine sexuality. Nor should Lacan's writings be divorced from the Ettingerian matrixial supplement. Indeed, Ettinger gives us much that is new and original in her formulation of the matrixial borderspace. Her writings are not only important to psychoanalysis and feminism but also to studies of sexuality, the maternal realm, and to the Feminine more broadly. But at the same time, something symptomatic, relating to knowledge and the Feminine, inclusive of the m/Other and the Woman occurs again. The whole truth can never be said as Lacan tells us. It is equally true that not all can be said with respect to Ettinger and Lacan.

In this book, I endeavor to interpret the theoretical convergence, alongside the impasse, between the two psychoanalytic scholars. Paradoxically, the impasse between Ettinger and Lacan enables something Real pertaining not only to knowledge, but to the Feminine and the m/Other, to emerge again: *Encore*.

Bibliography

Barzilai, Shuli. 1999. *Lacan and the Matter of Origins*. Stanford University Press.

Bollas, Christopher. 2006. Perceptive Identification. *The Psychoanalytic Review* (1963) (New York, NY) 93 (5): 713–17.

Buci-Glucksmann, Christine. 1996. Bracha Lichtenberg Ettinger: Images of Absence in the Inner Space of Painting. In *Inside the Visible: An Elliptical Traverse of 20th Century Art*, ed. Catherine de Zegher. The MIT Press.

Butler, Judith. 2004. Bracha's Eurydice. *Theory, Culture & Society* (London) 21 (1): 95–100. https://doi.org/10.1177/0263276404040481.

Butler, Judith. 2006. Bracha's Eurydice. In *The Matrixial Borderspace*, ed. Bracha Ettinger. University of Minnesota Press.

Caplan, Paula. 2002. *The New Don't Blame Mother: Mending the Mother-Daughter Relationship*. Routledge.

Cavanagh, Sheila. 2016. Tiresias and Psychoanalysis with/out Oedipus. *European Journal of Psychoanalysis* 28.

Cavanagh, Sheila. 2018. Bracha L. Ettinger, Jacques Lacan, and Tiresias: The Other Sexual Difference. *Sitegeist: A Journal for Psychoanalysis and Philosophy* 13:32–50.

Cavanagh, Sheila L. 2019. Tiresias: Bracha L. Ettinger and the Transgression with-in-to the Feminine. In *Femininity and Psychoanalysis*, ed. Agnieszka Piotrowska and Ben Tyrer, 1st ed. Routledge.
Cavanagh, Sheila. 2022. Tiresias and the Other Sexual Difference: Jacques Lacan and Bracha L. Ettinger. In *Psychoanalysis, Gender, and Sexualities: From Feminism to Trans*, ed. Patricia Gherovici and Manya Steinkoler. Cambridge University Press.
Copjec, Joan. 2004. *Imagine There's No Woman: Ethics and Sublimation*. The MIT Press.
Copjec, Joan. 2015. *Read My Desire: Lacan against the Historicists*, Radical Thinkers. Verso Books.
Ettinger, Bracha. 1996. Metramorphic Borderlinks and Matrixial Borderspace. In *Rethinking Borders*, ed. John C. Welchman. University of Minnesota Press.
Ettinger, Bracha. 1997. The Feminine/Prenatal Weaving in Matrixial Subjectivity-as-Encounter. *Psychoanalytic Dialogues* 7 (3): 367–405.
Ettinger, Bracha Lichtenberg. 2000. Transgressing With-In-To the Feminine. In *Differential Aesthetics: Art Practices, Philosophy and Feminist Understandings*, ed. Penny Florence and Nicola Foster, 1st ed. Routledge. https://doi.org/10.4324/9781315182735-13.
Ettinger, Bracha. 2001. Matrixial Gaze and Screen: Other Than Phallic and Beyond the Late Lacan. In *Bodies of Resistance: New Phenomenologies of Politics, Agency, and Culture*, ed. Laura Doyle. Northwestern University Press.
Ettinger, Bracha L. 2006a. Fascinance and the Girl-to-M/Other Matrixial Feminine Difference. In *Psychoanalysis and the Image*, ed. Griselda Pollock. Blackwell Publishing Ltd.
Ettinger, Bracha. 2006d. *The Matrixial Borderspace*, Theory out of Bounds. Vol. 28. University of Minnesota Press.
Ettinger, Bracha. 2010. Antigone With(out) Jocaste. In *Interrogating Antigone in Postmodern Philosophy and Criticism*, ed. Stephen Elliot Wilmer and Audrone Žukauskaitė. Oxford University Press.
Freud, Sigmund. 2017. *Three Essays on the Theory of Sexuality: The 1905 Edition*. Verso Books.
Grosz, Elizabeth. 2002. *Jacques Lacan: A Feminist Introduction*. Routledge.
Hirsch, Marianne. 1989. *The Mother Daughter Plot: Narrative, Psychoanalysis, Feminism*. Indiana University Press.
Janzen, Caitlin Audrey. 2022. "I'm Persephone, Queen of the Underworld": Metramorphic Swerves Away from Death in HBO's Sharp Objects. *Psychoanalysis, Culture & Society (London)* 27 (4): 502–521.

Kisiel, Anna. 2019. Aesth/Ethical Bodies: Bracha Ettinger's Eurydices and the Encounter With the Other's History. In *The Body in History, Culture, and the Arts*, ed. Aleksandra Musiał and Justyna Jajszczok, 1st ed. Routledge.

Kisiel, Anna. 2020. 'Gazing at Eurydice: Authorship and Otherness in Bracha L. *Ettinger'. Analyses/Rerearings/Theories (A/R/T) Journal* 6 (1): 7–17.

Lacan, Jacques. 1992. *The Ethics of Psychoanalysis 1959–1960: The Seminar of Jacques Lacan*. Edited by Jacques-Alain Miller. Translated by Dennis Porter. Book VII. W. W. Norton & Company Inc.

Lacan, Jacques. 1997. *The Seminar of Jacques Lacan: The Psychoses 1955–1956, Book III*. Reprint edition. Translated by Jacques-Alain Miller and Russell Grigg. Norton.

Lacan, Jacques. 1999. *On Feminine Sexuality: The Limits of Love and Knowledge*. In *On Feminine Sexuality: The Limits of Love and Knowledge*. Translated by Bruce Fink. The Seminar of Jacques Lacan. Norton.

Lacan, Jacques. 2002. *The Seminar of Jacques Lacan, Book XV: The Psychoanalytic Act, 1967–1968*. Translated by Cormac Gallagher. Karnac Books.

Lacan, Jacques. 2006a. Aggressiveness in Psychoanalysis. In *Écrits: The First Complete Edition in English*. Translated by Bruce Fink. W.W. Norton & Company.

Lacan, Jacques. 2006e. Guiding Remarks for a Conversation on Female Sexuality. In *Écrits: The First Complete Edition in English*. Translated by Bruce Fink. W.W. Norton & Company.

Lacan, Jacques. 2006f. Position of the Unconscious. In *Écrits: The First Complete Edition in English*. Translated by Bruce Fink. W.W. Norton & Company.

Lacan, Jacques. 2006g. The Subversion of the Subject and the Dialectic of Desire in the Freudian Unconscious. In *Écrits: The First Complete Edition in English*. Translated by Bruce Fink. W.W. Norton & Company.

Lacan, Jacques. 2006i. Psychoanalysis and Its Teaching. In *Écrits: The First Complete Edition in English*. Translated by Bruce Fink. W.W. Norton & Company.

Lacan, Jacques. 2006k. The Direction of the Treatment and the Principle of Its Power. In *Écrits: The First Complete Edition in English*. Translated by Bruce Fink. W.W. Norton & Company.

Lacan, Jacques. 2006o. On a Question Prior to Any Possible Treatment of Psychosis. In *Écrits: The First Complete Edition in English*. Translated by Bruce Fink. W.W. Norton & Company.

Lacan, Jacques. 2006p. On Freud's "Trieb" and the Psychoanalyst's Desire. In *Écrits: The First Complete Edition in English*. Translated by Bruce Fink. W.W. Norton & Company.

Lacan, Jacques. 2006q. The Youth of Gide, or the Letter and Desire. In *Écrits: The First Complete Edition in English*. Translated by Bruce Fink. W.W. Norton & Company.

Lacan, Jacques. 2018. *The Seminar of Jacques Lacan, Book XXIII: The Sinthome 1975–1976*. Edited by Jacques-Alain Miller. Translated by A. R. Price. Polity.

Lacan, Jacques. 2020. *The Seminar. Book IV: The Object Relation (1956–57)*. Edited by Jacques-Alain Miller. Translated by AR Price. Polity Press.

Mitchell, Juliet, and Jacqueline Rose. 1983. *Feminine Sexuality: Jacques Lacan and the École Freudienne*. Macmillan London.

Moi, Toril. 2004. From Femininity to Finitude: Freud, Lacan, and Feminism, Again. In *Dialogues on Sexuality, Gender, and Psychoanalysis*, ed. Iréne Matthis, 1st ed. Routledge.

Morel, Geneviève. 2019. *The Law of the Mother: An Essay on the Sexual Sinthome*. 1st ed. Routledge.

Pollock, Griselda. 2006. Femininity: Aporia or Sexual Difference? In *The Matrixial Borderspace*, Theory out of Bounds, ed. Bracha Ettinger, vol. 28. University of Minnesota Press.

Price, Adrian. 2008. Semblants and Sinthome in Freud's "Three Lines of Development". *Psychoanalytical Notebooks of the London Society of the New Lacanian School* 21:51–69.

Ragland-Sullivan, Ellie. 2012. *The Logic of Sexuation: From Aristotle to Lacan*, SUNY Series in Psychoanalysis and Culture. State University of New York Press.

Ragland-Sullivan, Ellie. 2014. The Sexual Masquerade: A Lacanian Theory of Sexual Difference. In *Lacan and the Subject of Language*, ed. Mark Bracher and Ellie Ragland-Sullivan, 1st ed. Routledge.

Rose, Jacqueline. 2005. *Sexuality in the Field of Vision*, Radical Thinkers. Vol. 9. Verso.

Schreber, Daniel Paul. 2000. *Memoirs of My Nervous Illness*. New York Review Books.

Smart, Genevieve. 2021. Impossible Births: Childbirth Beyond the (M)Other in Jacques Lacan and Mina Loy. *PSYART (Gainesville, Fla.)* (Gainesville), 1–1.

Soler, Colette. 2002. Hysteria in Scientific Discourse. In *Reading Seminar XX: Lacan's Major Work on Love, Knowledge, and Feminine Sexuality*, SUNY Series in Psychoanalysis and Culture, ed. Suzanne Barnard and Bruce Fink. State University of New York Press.

Soler, Colette. 2006. *What Lacan Said About Women: A Psychoanalytic Study*. Other Press, LLC.
Tsolas, Vaia. 2022. Misogyny, Mothers, Daughters and the Body. *Psychoanalytic Inquiry* (New York) 42 (7): 567–78.
Zupančič, Alenka. 2017. *What IS Sex?* Short Circuits. 1st ed. The MIT Press.

Bibliography

Abraham, Nicolas, and Maria Torok. 1994. *The Shell and the Kernel: Renewals of Psychoanalysis, Volume 1*. Translated by Nicholas T. Rand. Vol. 1. University of Chicago Press. WorldCat.

Baraitser, Lisa. 2013. Collecting Time: Some Reflections on the Psychopolitics of Belonging. *New Formations* (London) 79 (79): 8–25.

Baraitser, Lisa, Griselda Pollock, and Sigal Spigel. 2010. Editorial: M(O)Ther Trouble: Motherhood, Psychoanalysis, Feminism. Studies in the Maternal 2 (1). https://doi.org/10.16995/sim.80.

Barnard, Suzanne. 2002. Tongues of Angels: Feminine Structure and Other Jouissance. In *Reading Seminar XX: Lacan's Major Work on Love, Knowledge, and Feminine Sexuality*, ed. Suzanne Barnard and Bruce Fink. State University of New York Press.

Barzilai, Shuli. 1999. *Lacan and the Matter of Origins*. Stanford University Press.

Bertelsen, Lone. 2004. Matrixial Refrains. *Theory, Culture & Society* 21 (1): 121–147. https://doi.org/10.1177/0263276404040484.

Besdine, Matthew. 1968. The Jocasta Complex, Mothering and Genius, Part I. *Psychoanalytic Review* (New York) 55 (2): 259. 1310161122, p. 259. Periodicals Archive Online.

S. L. Cavanagh, *Bracha L. Ettinger and Jacques Lacan*, The Palgrave Lacan Series,
https://doi.org/10.1007/978-3-032-23293-9

Borossa, Julia, Catalina Bronstein, and Claire Pajaczkowska. 2015a. The New Dialogues: Freud, Klein, Lacan. In *The New Klein-Lacan Dialogues*. Taylor & Francis Group.

Borossa, Julia, Catalina Bronstein, and Claire Pajaczkowska. 2015b. The New Dialogues: Freud, Klein, Lacan. In *The New Klein-Lacan Dialogues*. Taylor & Francis Group.

Bourriaud, Nicolas. 2014. Bracha Ettinger: Off (Hors) Figures. *Image & Text: A Journal for Design* 23 (1): 18–33.

Brousse, Marie-Hélène. 2022. *The Feminine: A Mode of Jouissance*. Lacanian Press.

Butler, Judith. 1992. The Lesbian Phallus and the Morphological Imaginary. *Differences* 4 (1): 133–171.

Butler, Judith. 2002. *Antigone's Claim: Kinship between Life & Death*, The Wellek Library Lectures. Columbia University Press.

Butler, Judith. 2004a. *Precarious Life: The Powers of Mourning and Violence*. Verso.

Butler, Judith. 2004b. *Undoing Gender*. 1st ed. Taylor & Francis Group. https://doi.org/10.4324/9780203499627.

Butler, Judith. 2006. Bracha's Eurydice. In *The Matrixial Borderspace*, Theory out of Bounds, ed. Bracha Ettinger, vol. 28. University of Minnesota Press.

Butler, Judith. 2010. Promiscuous Obedience. In *Feminist Readings of Antigone*, ed. Fanny Söderbäck, 1st ed. State University of New York Press.

Butler, Judith. 2011. *Bodies That Matter: On the Discursive Limits of Sex*. Routledge.

Butler, Judith. 2016. *Frames of War: When Is Life Grievable?* Radical Thinkers. Verso.

Cavanagh, Sheila. 2016a. Tiresias and Psychoanalysis with/out Oedipus. *European Journal of Psychoanalysis* 28. Retrieved from http://www.journal-psychoanalysis.eu/

Cavanagh, Sheila L. 2016b. Transsexuality as Sinthome: Bracha L. Ettinger and the Other (Feminine) Sexual Difference. *Studies in Gender and Sexuality (Abingdon)* 17 (1): 27–44. https://doi.org/10.1080/15240657.2016.1135681.

Cavanagh, Sheila L. 2017. Antigone's legacy: A feminist psychoanalytic of an Other sexual difference. MAMSIE: *Studies in the Maternal*, 9(1), 4. http://doi.org/10.16995/sim.223.

Cavanagh, Sheila. 2018. Bracha L. Ettinger, Jacques Lacan, and Tiresias: The Other Sexual Difference. *Sitegeist: A Journal for Psychoanalysis and Philosophy* 13:32–50.

Cavanagh, Sheila L, 2019. Transgender, Hysteria, and the Other Sexual Difference: An Ettingerian Approach. *Studies in Gender and Sexuality* (Abingdon) 20 (1): 36–50. https://doi.org/10.1080/15240657.2019.1559517.

Cavanagh, Sheila L. 2019a. Tiresias: Bracha L. Ettinger and the Transgression with-in-to the Feminine. In *Femininity and Psychoanalysis*, ed. Agnieszka Piotrowska and Ben Tyrer, 1st ed. Routledge.

Cavanagh, Sheila L. 2019b. Transcryptums: An Ettingerian Reading of the Trans-Subjective Landscape in Transparent. *TSQ: Transgender Studies Quarterly* 6 (1): 20–42.

Cavanagh, Sheila, and Julián Daniel Gutiérrez-Albilla, eds. 2022. Special Issue: "The Psychoanalysis of Bracha L. Ettinger". *Psychoanalysis, Culture & Society*, Springer Nature.

Cavanagh, Sheila. 2022a. Tiresias and the Other Sexual Difference: Jacques Lacan and Bracha L. Ettinger. In *Psychoanalysis, Gender, and Sexualities: From Feminism to Trans*, ed. Patricia Gherovici and Manya Steinkoler. Cambridge University Press.

Cavanagh, Sheila L. 2022b. Transgender and the Other Sexual Difference in Vivek Shraya's Trisha. *Psychoanalysis, Culture & Society* (London) 27 (4): 485–501.

Cavanagh, Sheila L. 2023. The Matrixial Gaze: Transgender in Boys Don't Cry. *Studies in Gender and Sexuality* (Abingdon) 23 (4): 243–55.

Cavanagh, Sheila, and Julián Daniel Gutiérrez-Albilla, eds. n.d. Special Issue: "The Psychoanalysis of Bracha L. Ettinger". *Psychoanalysis, Culture & Society* 27 (4).

Cejudo-Escamilla, Sonia. 2021. Trauma and Transcryptum: Towards a Feminist Methodology for the Analysis of Narratives of Trauma. *Sociología y Tecnociencia* 11 (1): 104–124.

Cixous, Hélène. 2009. The Laugh of the Medusa. In *Feminisms Redux: An Anthology of Literary Theory and Criticism*, ed. Robyn R. Warhol and Diane Price Herndl. Rutgers University Press.

Copjec, Joan. 2002. *UMBR(a): A Journal of the Unconscious*. UMBR(a).

Copjec, Joan. 2004a. *Imagine There's No Woman: Ethics and Sublimation*. The MIT Press. https://doi.org/10.7551/mitpress/3668.001.0001.

Copjec, Joan. 2004b. *Imagine There's No Woman: Ethics and Sublimation*. The MIT Press.

Copjec, Joan. 2015. *Read My Desire: Lacan against the Historicists*, Radical Thinkers. Verso Books.

Copjec, Joan. 2018. The Sexual Compact. In *Sex and Nothing*, ed. Alejandro Cerda-Rueda, 1st ed. Routledge.

Daly, Ruth. 2021. Disrupting Phallic Logic: (Re)Thinking the Feminine with Hélène Cixous and Bracha Ettinger. *Australian Feminist Studies* (ABINGDON) 36 (109): 335–51.

Deleuze, Gilles, and Félix Guattari. 1987. Introduction. In *A Thousand Plateaus Capitalism and Schizophrenia*. University of Minnesota Press.

Duras, Marguerite. 1966. *The Ravishing of Lol Stein*. Translated by Richard Seaver. Grove Press.

Duras, Marguerite. 1967. *The Sea Wall (Un Barrage Contre Le Pacifique)*. Translated by Herma Briffault. Farrar, Straus and Giroux.

Duras, Marguerite. 2019. Motherhood Makes You Obscene. *The Paris Review*, October 1. https://www.theparisreview.org/blog/2019/10/01/motherhood-makes-you-obscene/.

Ettinger, Bracha Lichtenberg. 1992. Matrix and Metramorphosis. *Differences: A Journal of Feminist Cultural Studies* 4 (3): 176–209.

Ettinger, Bracha. 1993. *Matrix Halal (a): Lapsus: Notes on Painting*. Museum of modern art.

Ettinger, Bracha. 1994. The Becoming Threshold of Matrixial Borderlines. In *Travellers' Tales: Narratives of Home and Displacement*, ed. George Robertson, Melinda Mash, Lisa Tickner, Jon Bird, Barry Curtis, and Tim Putnam. Routledge.

Ettinger, Bracha. 1996. Metramorphic Borderlinks and Matrixial Borderspace. In *Rethinking Borders*, ed. John C. Welchman. University of Minnesota Press.

Ettinger, Bracha. 1997. The Feminine/Prenatal Weaving in Matrixial Subjectivity-as-Encounter. *Psychoanalytic Dialogues* 7 (3): 367–405.

Ettinger, Bracha. 2000a. Art as the Transport-Station of Trauma. In *Bracha Lichtenberg Ettinger: Artworking, 1985–1999*. Ludion: Palais des Beaux-Arts.

Ettinger, Bracha Lichtenberg. 2000c. Transgressing With-In-To the Feminine. In *Differential Aesthetics: Art Practices, Philosophy and Feminist Understandings*, ed. Penny Florence and Nicola Foster, 1st ed. Routledge. https://doi.org/10.4324/9781315182735-13.

Ettinger, Bracha. 2001aa. Matrixial Gaze and Screen: Other Than Phallic and Beyond the Late Lacan. In *Bodies of Resistance: New Phenomenologies of Politics, Agency, and Culture*, ed. Laura Doyle. Northwestern University Press.

Ettinger, Bracha. 2001ab. Matrixial Gaze and Screen: Other Than Phallic and Beyond the Late Lacan. In *Bodies of Resistance: New Phenomenologies of Politics, Agency, and Culture*, ed. Laura Doyle. Northwestern University Press.

Ettinger, Bracha Lichtenberg. 2001b. The Red Cow Effect: The Metramorphosis of Hallowing the Hollow and Hollowing the Hallow. In *He Said, She Says: An RSVP to the Male Text*, ed. Mica Howe and Sarah Appleton Aguiar. Fairleigh Dickinson University Press.

Ettinger, Bracha. 2002a. From Transference to the Aesthetic Paradigm: A Conversation with Félix Guattari. In *A Shock to Thought: Expression after Deleuze and Guattari*, ed. Brian Massumi. Routledge.

Ettinger, Bracha Lichtenberg. 2002b. Trans-Subjective Transferential Borderspace. In *A Shock to Thought: Expression after Deleuze and Guattari*. Routledge.

Ettinger, Bracha. 2004. Weaving a Woman Artist With-in the Matrixial Encounter-Event. *Theory, Culture & Society* 21 (1): 69–94.

Ettinger, Bracha. 2005. Copoiesis. *Ephemera: Theory & Politics in Organization* 5 (X): 703–713.

Ettinger, Bracha L. 2006a. Fascinance and the Girl-to-M/Other Matrixial Feminine Difference. In *Psychoanalysis and the Image*, ed. Griselda Pollock. Blackwell Publishing Ltd.

Ettinger, Bracha. 2006b. From Proto-Ethical Compassion to Responsibility: Besideness and the Three Primal Mother-Phantasies of Not-Enoughness, Devouring and Abandonment. *Athena* 1 (2): 100–135.

Ettinger, Bracha. 2006c. Matrixial Trans-Subjectivity. *Theory, Culture & Society* (London, Thousand Oaks, CA and New Delhi) 23 (2–3): 218–22.

Ettinger, Bracha. 2006d. *The Matrixial Borderspace*, Theory out of Bounds. Vol. 28. University of Minnesota Press.

Ettinger, Bracha Lichtenberg. 2007. Diotima and the Matrixial Transference: Psychoanalytical Encounter-Event as Pregnancy in Beauty. In *Beyond the Threshold: Explorations of Liminality in Literature*, ed. Hein Viljoen and N. Chris. Van der Merwe. Peter Lang.

Ettinger, Bracha Lichtenberg. 2009a. Fragilization and Resistance. *Studies in the Maternal* 1 (2): 1–31. https://doi.org/10.16995/sim.141.

Ettinger, Bracha Lichtenberg. 2009b. "Fragilization and Resistance" and "Neighborhood and Shechina". *Studies in the Maternal* 1 (2): 1–31. https://doi.org/10.16995/sim.141.

Ettinger, Bracha. 2010. Antigone With(out) Jocaste. In *Interrogating Antigone in Postmodern Philosophy and Criticism*, ed. Stephen Elliot Wilmer and Audrone Žukauskaitė. Oxford University Press.

Ettinger, Bracha Lichtenberg. 2016. Laius Complex and Shocks of Maternality: With Franz Kafka and Sylvia Plath. In *Interdisciplinary Handbook of Trauma and Culture*, ed. Haviva Pedaya, David Gurevitz, Yuval Neria, and Yochai Ataria. Springer International Publishing.

Ettinger, B. 2019. Beyond the Death-Drive, beyond the Life-Drive: Being-toward-Birthing with Being-toward-Birth; Copoiesis and the Matrixial Eros—Metafeminist Notes. In *Aberrant Nuptials: Deleuze and Artistic Research*, 183–214. Leuven University Press.

Fink, Bruce. 2002. Knowledge and Jouissance. In *Reading Seminar XX: Lacan's Major Work on Love, Knowledge, and Feminine Sexuality*, ed. Suzanne Barnard and Bruce Fink. State University of New York Press.

Fisher, R. Michael. 2024. Teaching Ettingerian Matrixial Theory. *Artizein: Arts and Teaching Journal* 9 (1): 12.

Freeland, Charles. 2013. *Antigone, in Her Unbearable Splendor: New Essays on Jacques Lacan's The Ethics of Psychoanalysis*. State University of New York Press.

Freud, Sigmund. 1963. *Dora: An Analysis of a Case of Hysteria*. 1997th ed. Simon and Schuster.

Giffney, Noreen, Anne Mulhall, and Michael O'Rourke. 2009. Seduction into Reading: Bracha L. Ettinger's The Matrixial Borderspace. *Studies in the Maternal* 1(2): 1–15. https://doi.org/10.16995/sim.140.

Grosz, Elizabeth. 2002. *Jacques Lacan: A Feminist Introduction*. Routledge.

Grosz, Elizabeth. 2017. Psychoanalysis and the Body. In *Feminist Theory and the Body*. Routledge.

Grosz, Elizabeth. 2020a. *Sexual Subversions*. Routledge.

Grosz, Elizabeth. 2020b. *Volatile Bodies*. Routledge.

Gutiérrez-Albilla, Julián Daniel. 2022. Introduction: The Primary Event of Peace: Femininity, Com-Passionate Hospitality, and Aesthetic Wit(h)Nessing in Bracha L. Ettinger's Matrixial Psychoanalysis. *Psychoanalysis, Culture & Society* (London) 27 (4): 466–84.

Haruki, Namiko. 2012. Ab-Sense of Existence in "The Ravishing of Lol Stein" by Marguerite Duras. *PSYART: A Hyperlink Journal for the Psychological Study of the Arts*, 5.

Honig, Bonnie. 2011. Ismene's Forced Choice: Sacrifice and Sorority in Sophocles. *Antigone'. Arethusa* 44 (1): 29–68.

Irigaray, Luce. 2010. The Eternal Irony of the Community. In *Feminist Readings of Antigone*, SUNY Series in Gender Theory, ed. Fanny Söderbäck. SUNY Press.

Johnson, Anna Louise. 2006. Bracha Ettinger's Theory of the Matrix: Contexts and Commentary. ProQuest Dissertations & Theses.

Johnston, Adrian. 2019. Lacan's Endgame: Philosophy, Science, and Religion in the Final Seminars. *Crisis and Critique* 6 (1): 157–187.

Kinsella, Tina. 2019. A Cord That Is Never Done Away with: An Aesthetic Ontology of the Pre-Birth Scene with Francesca Woodman and Bracha L. Ettinger. In *Maternal Structures in Art: Intergenerational Discussions on Motherhood and Creative Work*, ed. Valerie Walkerdine and Elena Marchevska, 1st ed. Routledge.

Kisiel, Anna. 2017. Dis-obedience to the Father Bracha L. Ettinger's Theory and Installation Confronted with Freud and Lacan. *Romanica Silesiana* 12:53–63.

Kisiel, Anna. 2019. Aesth/Ethical Bodies: Bracha Ettinger's Eurydices and the Encounter With the Other's History. In *The Body in History, Culture, and the Arts*, ed. Aleksandra Musiał and Justyna Jajszczok, 1st ed. Routledge.

Kisiel, Anna. 2020. 'Gazing at Eurydice: Authorship and Otherness in Bracha L. Ettinger. *Analyses/Rerearings/Theories (A/R/T) Journal* 6 (1): 7–17.

Kisiel, Anna. 2022. Openness in Distance: Introductory Remarks on Academic Teaching Informed by Bracha L. Ettinger's Matrixial Theory. *Studies in Philosophy and Education (Dordrecht)* 41 (5): 497–509.

Kristeva, J. 1973. The Semiotic Activity. *Screen (London)* (London) 14 (1–2): 25–39.

Kristeva, Julia. 1980. *Desire in Language: A Semiotic Approach to Literature and Art*, European Perspectives. Columbia University Press.

Kristeva, Julia. 1982. *Powers of Horror: An Essay on Abjection*, European Perspectives. Vol. 98. Columbia University Press.

Kristeva, Julia. 2002. *Intimate Revolt*, European Perspectives: A Series in Social Thought and Cultural Criticism Series. Vol. v, 2. Columbia University Press. https://books.google.ca/books?id=xq2MLJAw8koC.

Kristeva, Julia. 2010. Limit and Horizon. In *Feminist Readings of Antigone*, ed. Fanny Söderbäck, 1st ed. State University of New York Press.

Lacan, Jacques. 1981. *Les Non-Dupes Errent.*

Lacan, Jacques. 1987. Homage to Marguerite Duras, on Le Ravissement de Lol V. Stein. In *Marguerite Duras*. Translated by Peter Connor. City Lights Books.

Lacan, Jacques. 1992. *The Ethics of Psychoanalysis 1959–1960: The Seminar of Jacques Lacan*. Edited by Jacques-Alain Miller. Translated by Dennis Porter. Book VII. W. W. Norton & Company Inc.

Lacan, Jacques. 1997. *The Seminar of Jacques Lacan: The Psychoses 1955–1956, Book III*. Reprint edition. Translated by Jacques-Alain Miller and Russell Grigg. Norton.

Lacan, Jacques. 1998a. *The Seminar of Jacques Lacan, Book XX: On Feminine Sexuality: The Limits of Love and Knowledge (Encore 1972–1973)*. Edited by Jacques-Alain Miller and Bruce Fink. WW Norton & Company.

Lacan, Jacques. 1998b. *The Four Fundamental Concepts of Psychoanalysis, The Seminar of Jacques Lacan, Book XI*. Edited by Jacques-Alain Miller. Translated by Alan Sheridan. WW Norton & Company.

Lacan, Jacques. 2006. *Écrits: The First Complete Edition in English*. Translated by Bruce Fink. W.W. Norton & Company.

Lacan, Jacques. 2006e. Guiding Remarks for a Conversation on Female Sexuality. In *Écrits: The First Complete Edition in English*. Translated by Bruce Fink. W.W. Norton & Company.

Lacan, Jacques. 2006f. Position of the Unconscious. In *Écrits: The First Complete Edition in English*. Translated by Bruce Fink. W.W. Norton & Company.

Lacan, Jacques. 2006j. A Theoretical Introduction to the Functions of Psychoanalysis in Criminology. In *Écrits: The First Complete Edition in English*. Translated by Bruce Fink. W.W. Norton & Company.

Lacan, Jacques. 2006m. Introduction to Jean Hyppolite's Commentary on Freud's Verneinung. In *Écrits: The First Complete Edition in English*. Translated by Bruce Fink, vols 308–317. W.W. Norton & Company.

Lacan, Jacques. 2006ba. Presentation on Psychic Causality. In *Écrits: The First Complete Edition in English*. Translated by Bruce Fink. W.W. Norton & Company.

Lacan, Jacques. 2006bb. Presentation on Psychic Causality. In *Écrits: The First Complete Edition in English*. Translated by Bruce Fink. W.W. Norton & Company.

Lacan, Jacques. 2006c. Remarks on Daniel Lagache's Presentation: "Psychoanalysis and Personality Structure. In *Écrits: The First Complete Edition in English*. Translated by Bruce Fink. W.W. Norton & Company.

Lacan, Jacques. 2006d. Response to Jean Hyppolite's Commentary on Freud's "Verneinung". In *Écrits: The First Complete Edition in English*. Translated by Bruce Fink. W.W. Norton & Company.

Lacan, Jacques. 2006g. The Subversion of the Subject and the Dialectic of Desire in the Freudian Unconscious. In *Écrits: The First Complete Edition in English*. Translated by Bruce Fink. W.W. Norton & Company.

Lacan, Jacques. 2006h. Presentation on Transference. In *Écrits: The First Complete Edition in English*. Translated by Bruce Fink. W.W. Norton & Company.

Lacan, Jacques. 2006i. Psychoanalysis and Its Teaching. In *Écrits: The First Complete Edition in English*. Translated by Bruce Fink. W.W. Norton & Company.

Lacan, Jacques. 2006l. The Function and Field of Speech and Language in Psychoanalysis. In *Écrits: The First Complete Edition in English*. Translated by Bruce Fink. W.W. Norton & Company.

Lacan, Jacques. 2011. The Seminar of Jacques Lacan: Book X: Anxiety: 1962–1963. Unpublished manuscript. Translated by Cormac Gallagher.

Lacan, Jacques. 2014. *The Seminar of Jacques Lacan, Book X: Anxiety*. Edited by Jacques-Alain Miller. Translated by AR Price. Polity Press.

Lacan, Jacques. 2018. *The Seminar of Jacques Lacan, Book XXIII: The Sinthome 1975–1976*. Edited by Jacques-Alain Miller. Translated by A. R. Price. Polity.

Lacan, Jacques. 2020. *The Seminar. Book IV: The Object Relation (1956–57)*. Edited by Jacques-Alain Miller. Translated by AR Price. Polity Press.

MacNamara, Nóirín. 2021. Precarity and Judith Butler's Ambivalent Social Bond. What Is the Value of Ettingerian Transconnectedness? *Precarity and International Relations*, 203–28.

MacNamara, Nóirín. 2024. The Value of Owning the Symbols That Orientate Us within Subjectivity. *Feminist Theory* (London, England) 26 (2): 426–45.

Malone, Kareen Ror. 1997. Working through the Question of the Phallus to the Other Side Commentary on Bracha Lichtenberg-Ettinger's Paper. *Psychoanalytic Dialogues* 7 (3): 407–422.

Massumi, Brian. 2006. Painting: The Voice of the Grain. In *The Matrixial Borderspace*, Theory out of Bounds, ed. Bracha Ettinger, vol. 28. University of Minnesota Press.

Miller, Paul Allen. 2013. Duras and Platonic Love: The Erotics of Substitution. *The Comparatist* 37 (1): 83–104.

Millot, Catherine. 1990. *Horsexe: Essay on Transsexuality*. Autonomedia.

Mitchell, Juliet, and Jacqueline Rose. 1983. *Feminine Sexuality: Jacques Lacan and the École Freudienne*. Macmillan London.

Morel, Geneviève. 2002. Feminine Conditions of Jouissance. In *Reading Seminar XX: Lacan's Major Work on Love, Knowledge, and Feminine Sexuality*, ed. Suzanne Barnard and Bruce Fink. State University of New York Press.

Morel, Genevieve. 2011. *Sexual Ambiguities: Sexuation and Psychosis*. Centre for Freudian Analysis and Research Library. Karnac Books.

Morel, Geneviève. 2018. *The Law of the Mother: An Essay on the Sexual Sinthome*. 1st ed. Routledge.

Neill, Calum. 2008. Severality: Beyond the Compression of the Cogito. *Subjectivity* 24 (1): 325–339. https://doi.org/10.1057/sub.2008.21.

Pollock, Griselda. 1992. 'Trouble in the Archives: Introduction'. *Differences: A Journal of Feminist. Cultural Studies* 4 (3): iii–xiv.

Pollock, Griselda. 1994. The Work of Bracha Lichtenberg-Ettinger: An Introduction. *Third Text (London)* 8 (28–29): 61–70.

Pollock, Griselda. 1996. "Gleaning in History or Coming After/behind the Reapers: The Feminine, the Stranger and the Matrix in the Work and Theory of Bracha Lichtenberg Ettinger." In Generations and Geographies in the Visual Arts: Feminist Readings, edited by Griselda Pollock, 342–73. London: Routledge.

Pollock, Griselda. 1999. Painting as a Backward Glance That Does Not Kill: Eurydice (1992–99) by Bracha Lichtenberg Ettinger. *Renaissance and Modern Studies* 42 (1): 116–144.

Pollock, Griselda. 2004. Thinking the Feminine: Aesthetic Practice as Introduction to Bracha Ettinger and the Concepts of Matrix and Metramorphosis. *Theory, Culture & Society* (London) 21 (1): 5–65.

Pollock, Griselda. 2005. Gleaning in History or Coming after/behind the Reapers: The Feminine, the Stranger and the Matrix in the Work and Theory of Bracha Lichtenberg Ettinger. In *Generations and Geographies in the Visual Arts: Feminist Readings*. Routledge.

Pollock, Griselda. 2006. Femininity: Aporia or Sexual Difference? In *The Matrixial Borderspace*, Theory out of Bounds, ed. Bracha Ettinger, vol. 28. University of Minnesota Press.

Pollock, Griselda. 2007. What Does a Woman Want? Art Investigating Death in Charlotte Salomon's Leben? Oder Theater? *Art History* (Oxford, UK) 30 (3): 383–405.

Pollock, Griselda. 2009a. Art/Trauma/Representation. *Parallax (Leeds, England)* (ABINGDON) 15 (1): 40–54.

Pollock, Griselda. 2009b. Mother Trouble: The Maternal-Feminine in Phallic and Feminist Theory in Relation to Bratta Ettinger's Elaboration of Matrixial Ethics. *Studies in the Maternal* 1 (1): 1–31.

Pollock, Griselda. 2013. Art as Transport-Station of Trauma? Haunting Objects in the Works of Bracha Ettinger, Sarah Kofman and Chantal Akerman. In *Representing Auschwitz: At the Margins of Testimony*. Springer.

Pollock, Griselda. 2014a. Abandoned at the Mouth of Hell or a Second Look That Does Not Kill: The Uncanny Coming to Matrixial Memory. In *Looking Back to the Future*, ed. Saul Ostrow, 1st ed. Routledge.

Pollock, Griselda. 2014b. Sarah Kofman's Father's Pen and Bracha Ettinger's Mother's Spoon: Trauma, Transmission and the Strings of Virtuality. In *Objects and Materials*, ed. Gillian Evans, Penny Harvey, Elizabeth B. Silva, et al., 1st ed. Routledge.

Pollock, Griselda. 2016. Is Feminism a Trauma, a Bad Memory, or a Virtual Future? *Differences* 27 (2): 27–61.

Pollock, Griselda. 2017. The Missing Wit(h)Ness: Monroe, Fascinance and the Unguarded Intimacy of Being Dead. *Journal of Visual Art Practice* 16 (3): 265–296.

Pollock, Griselda. 2019. "Akerman" on-Screen: Chantal Akerman behind and before the Camera, and after Cinema. *Moving Image Review & Art Journal* 8 (1–2): 8–26.

Pollock, Griselda. 2023a. *Encounters in the Virtual Feminist Museum: Time, Space and the Archive*. Routledge.

Pollock, Griselda. 2023b. The Graces of Catastrophe: Matrixial Time and Aesthetic Space Confront the Archive of Disaster. In *Encounters in the Virtual Feminist Museum*. Routledge.

Pollok, Griselda. 2006. Beyond Oedipus: Feminist Thought, Psychoanalysis and Mythical Figurations of the Feminine. In *Laughing with Medusa: Classical Myth and Feminist Thought*, Classical Presences, ed. Vando Zajko and Miriam Leonard. Oxford University Press. https://doi.org/10.1093/acprof:oso/9780199237944.001.0001.

Rabaté, Jean-Michel. 2019. Falling in Love with Marguerite Duras. *Journal of the Circle for Lacanian Ideology Critique* 12:5–14.

Ragland, Ellie. 2008. The Masquerade, the Veil, and the Phallic Mask. *Psychoanalysis, Culture & Society (London)* 13 (1): 8–23.

Ragland-Sullivan, Ellie. 2012. *The Logic of Sexuation: From Aristotle to Lacan*, SUNY Series in Psychoanalysis and Culture. State University of New York Press.

Ragland-Sullivan, Ellie. 2014. The Sexual Masquerade: A Lacanian Theory of Sexual Difference. In *Lacan and the Subject of Language*, ed. Mark Bracher and Ellie Ragland-Sullivan, 1st ed. Routledge.

Rank, Otto. 2015. *The Trauma of Birth*. Ravenio Books.

Rodriguez, Karen. 2016. Someone Else Is Singing through Your Throat: Language, Trauma and Bracha L. Ettinger's Wit (h) Nessing. *Critical Multilingualism Studies* 4 (1): 25–43.

Rose, Jacqueline. 2005. *Sexuality in the Field of Vision*, Radical Thinkers. Vol. 9. Verso.

Rowley, Alison. 1999. An Introduction to Bracha Lichtenberg-Ettinger's Traumatic Wit(h)Ness-Thing and Matrixial Co/in-Habit(u)Ating. *Parallax (Leeds, England)* 5 (1): 83–88.

Sander, Nina. 2024. Heartbreak and Wild Possibilities: Sublime Encounters with the Eco-Maternal. *Psychoanalytic Perspectives* 21 (3): 373–393.

Schilder, Paul. 2013. *The Image and Appearance of the Human Body*. Routledge.

Silverman, Kaja. 1992. The Lacanian Phallus. *Differences* 4 (1): 84–115.

Simon, Tracy. 2024. Mothers: Inhabiting the Impossible. *Studies in Gender and Sexuality (Abingdon)* 25 (3): 191–198.

Sjöholm, Cecilia. 2004. *The Antigone Complex: Ethics and the Invention of Feminine Desire*. 1st ed. Stanford University Press.

Smart, Genevieve. 2021. Impossible Births: Childbirth Beyond the (M)Other in Jacques Lacan and Mina Loy. *PSYART (Gainesville, Fla.)* (Gainesville), 1–1.

Smith, Mariëlle. 2013. Subjectivity as Encounter: Feminine Ethics in the Work of Bracha Lichtenberg-Ettinger and Anne Enright. *Hypatia* (HOBOKEN) 28 (3): 633–45.

Söderbäck, Fanny, ed. 2010. *Feminist Readings of Antigone*, SUNY Series in Gender Theory. SUNY Press.

Soler, Colette. 2002. Hysteria in Scientific Discourse. In *Reading Seminar XX: Lacan's Major Work on Love, Knowledge, and Feminine Sexuality*, SUNY Series in Psychoanalysis and Culture, ed. Suzanne Barnard and Bruce Fink. State University of New York Press.

Soler, Colette. 2002b. What Does the Unconscious Know About Women. In *Reading Seminar XX: Lacan's Major Work on Love, Knowledge, and Feminine Sexuality*, SUNY Series in Psychoanalysis and Culture, ed. Suzanne Barnard and Bruce Fink. State University of New York Press.

Soler, Colette. 2006a. *What Lacan Said About Women: A Psychoanalytic Study*. Other Press, LLC.

Soler, Colette. 2006b. *What Lacan Said about Women: A Psychoanalytic Study*. Translated by John Holland. Other Press.

Soler, Colette. 2012. Identité et sexuation. In *Désirs et sexualités*. Érès.

Soler, Colette. 2023. *Towards Identity in the Psychoanalytic Encounter: A Lacanian Perspective*. 1st ed. Routledge.

Soler, Colette, and Bruce Fink. 2015. *Lacanian Affects: The Function of Affect in Lacan's Work*. Routledge.

Solstreif-Pirker, Christoph. 2022. The Scream Is Not Silenced: A Mountainous Passage to Ettingerian Environmental Ethics. *Psychoanalysis, Culture & Society* (London) 27 (4): 563–78.

Solstreif-Pirker, Christoph. 2023. Toward a Feminine-Matrixial Understanding of Modernity: Subjectivity-as-World-Fabric, the Ecology of Love, and the Temporality of Just Now. *Comparative Literature Studies (Urbana)* (UNIVERSITY PK) 60 (3): 561–77.

Sophocles. 1984. *The Three Theban Plays: Antigone, Oedipus the King, Oedipus at Colonus*. Translated by Robert Fagles. Penguin Classics.

Torre, Shanna de la. 2018. *Sex for Structuralists: The Non-Oedipal Logics of Femininity and Psychosis*. Palgrave Macmillan.

Van Loo, Sofie. 2009. Colourline painting by Bracha L. Ettinger: the transject as abstract-realist artwork in an analogue-dialogue with the (un) heimliche. *Studies in the Maternal* 1(2): 1–10. https://doi.org/10.16995/sim.143.

Vigneault, Marissa. 2011. The Porous Space of Bracha Ettinger's Eurydices. In *Contemporary Art and Classical Myth*, 111–133. Ashgate Publishing, Ltd.

Voela, Angie. 2014. Wit (h) Finessing the Other's Trauma. In *The Ethics of Remembering and the Consequences of Forgetting: Essays on Trauma, History, and Memory*, New Imago: Series in Theoretical, Clinical, and Applied Psychoanalysis, ed. Michael O'Loughlin. Rowman & Littlefield.

Voela, Angie, and Cigdem Esin. 2021. Movement, Embrace: Adriana Cavarero with Bracha Lichtenberg Ettinger (and the Death Drive). *Hypatia* (NEW YORK) 36 (1): 101–19.

Voruz, Véronique. 2007. A Lacanian Reading of Dora. In *The Later Lacan: An Introduction*, ed. Véronique Voruz and Bogdan Wolf. State University of New York Press.

Walsh, Fintan. 2011. From Enthusiasm to Encounter-Event: Bracha L. Ettinger, Samuel Beckett and the Theatre of Affect. *Parallax (Leeds, England)* (ABINGDON) 17 (2): 110–23.

Wierzchowska, Justyna. 2022. Creating Together an "Unexpected Home": Navigating the Matrixial Borderspace Through Text and Image in Mary Kelly's Post-Partum Document (1973–79). In *Text and Image in Women's Life Writing*, Palgrave Studies in Life Writing, ed. Stephanie Genty, Nicoleta Alexoae-Zagni, Corinne Bigot, Claire Bazin, and Valérie Baisnée-Keay. Springer International Publishing.

Zajko, Vanda, and Miriam Leonard, eds. 2006. *Laughing with Medusa: Classical Myth and Feminist Thought*. OUP Oxford.

Zupančič, Alenka. 2017. *What is Sex?* Short Circuits. 1st ed. The MIT Press.

Index[1]

[1] Note: Page numbers followed by 'n' refer to notes.

S. L. Cavanagh, *Bracha L. Ettinger and Jacques Lacan*, The Palgrave Lacan Series,
https://doi.org/10.1007/978-3-032-23293-9

G

H

I

J

K

L

M

FSC
www.fsc.org
MIX
Papier | Fördert gute Waldnutzung
FSC® C083411

Kolibri 360 GmbH
Ferdinand-Jühlke-Straße 7
99095 Erfurt, Deutschland
produktsicherheit@kolibri360.de